STOP SMOKING!

STOP SMOKING!

BEATING NICOTINE ADDICTION

RENÉE BITTOUN

RANDOM HOUSE
AUSTRALIA

Random House Australia Pty Ltd
20 Alfred Street, Milsons Point, NSW 2061

Sydney New York Toronto
London Auckland
and agencies throughout the world

First published 1993

National Library of Australia
Cataloguing-in-Publication Data

Bittoun, Renée.
  Stop smoking!

  ISBN 0 09 182795 7.

  1. Cigarette smokers – Rehabilitation. 2. Tobacco
  habit – Treatment. 3. Self-help techniques. I. Title.

613.85

Typeset by Midland Typesetters, Victoria
Printed by Griffin Paperbacks, Adelaide
Production by Vantage Graphics, Sydney

CONTENTS

Dedication

In memory of my grandparents

Acknowledgements

I am grateful firstly to John Mangos for initiating this project, to Greg Smith for assisting with the draft and to Dr Karl-Olov Fagerström for permission to use his questionnaire. Thanks also go to my colleagues Dr Chris Clarke, Dr Peter Maloney, Joy Petrie and Diane Kingsford-Archer for reviewing the manuscript and finally to Professor David Bryant for his support and encouragement over many years.

INTRODUCTION

Why is it that so many smokers find it difficult to quit? So many smokers have undergone the dilemma of wishing to quit, and then been unsuccessful so it seems obvious that there must be more to their smoking than just a bad habit.

Why would anyone want to go on smoking today? The evidence that it is unhealthy is overwhelming. Socially it's unacceptable and it costs too much. It's written on the box that it might kill you, yet a lot of people persist in smoking despite all of this. Most people who smoke are sane and rational but for some reason they have no control over their smoking. It's often a love–hate relationship. Some really enjoy it but may feel secretly they have a suicidal bent or that they have no willpower, that they are weak or have an addictive personality. Some smokers are labelled by others as fools with no backbone who don't understand the implications of what they are doing. The pressure to quit smoking in our society today is very strong. Not only do children harangue their parents about it, couples break up because of it. The issue of passive smoking too has polarised the community, antagonising smokers who are insistent that it is a question of their civil rights.

So why the difficulty in quitting? Few smokers ever perceive their smoking has become a question of dependence or addiction. If they do so, the words are used with little comprehension of what an addiction actually implies. The idea often horrifies smokers, who feel they might be put in the same category as drug addicts and can't accept this concept.

After years of experience with smokers wishing to quit it has become evident that smoking is not simply a bad habit. The word habit itself should be stricken from the lexicon of smoking, for it is far from that. All addictions or dependencies are manifested by withdrawals, tolerance and relapse; and smoking falls precisely into this category. No 'mind set' or mental decision on the part of the addicted smoker will change this. Today enough scientific evidence has been collected to begin to explain why some smokers have had such difficulties with quitting. No matter how intellectually astute an addicted smoker may be, no amount of rationalisation will be able to curtail their craving for a cigarette. Neither IQ nor education has anything to do with addiction. Nor does sex, age or socio-economic status. It cannot be ignored that smokers receive many positive effects from smoking, which enhances their continuing need to smoke.

This book is aimed at giving an informed and intelligent approach to smoking and its causes. Can simply reading a book about smoking help you quit? A newer, more sympathetic and objective look at smoking is presented here. A perspective perhaps that will lead to a better approach in affecting a change. There is no point in berating someone who smokes when they obviously have little or no control over it. Accordingly there is little in this book about the ill effects of smoking, but more on the actual activity. It guides on the best methods to ultimately deal with the addiction and maintenance of abstinence.

If you have bought this book for yourself with the aim to do something about your smoking, you have already made a major decision towards that change, but how is it possible to convince someone else to read this book? I have often been confronted with a situation where a friend, a wife, a husband or parent has begged me to talk their smoking loved one into doing something about it. This is the hardest part of all quitting. Information and ideas, love and deep concern on the part of others are not enough. *The person must want to stop.* They will undoubtedly claim they've heard it all before, and they are right. There is always the newest 'magic bullet' on the market. We can only now be more understanding and sympathetic to the smoker, with what we know about nicotine dependency today. Assuring a smoker that this book is not about 'how bad smoking is for your health' may be one way of convincing them to take a look.

In nearly every smoker there is the ambivalence—the love–hate relationship with their smoking, and many smokers simply like doing it. 'Why should I quit? I like it.' There is no denying that smokers enjoy their smoking because of the myriad of positive psychological effects it can give them, despite what they know of the negative physical effects. Ultimately no amount of cajoling is going to help; it may even be counterproductive. Motivation to change a behaviour comes from within over stages. But sometimes it can be an acute event, like an asthma attack, that can trigger off the desire for an immediate change; and sometimes it's a long slow thought process that's taken years to mull over. The information presented in this book may add to the accumulated knowledge that a smoker may already have and be just that extra trigger that sets in motion a step towards behavioural changes.

At the beginning of this century manufactured cigarettes began to cover the globe and in their wake came millions of nicotine addicts. With the advent of personal freedom and liberty that is now sweeping the world towards the end of this century it is, however, timely that all smokers liberate themselves from the tyranny of nicotine addiction.

⊗ 1 ⊗

NICOTINE: THE ADDICTION

Over the past ten years there has been a wealth of research carried out on the topic of why people smoke. We know that what influences a young person to start to smoke is not the same reason they continue to do so into adulthood. The initiation into smoking is a complex social phenomenon with much of its basis in peer-group pressure, social norms and advertising. These can also be the same reasons people wish to quit. There is strong peer-group pressure in the older age groups for non-smoking, socially there are less and less venues to be able to smoke freely, and the anti-smoking advertising campaigns have taken their toll on ambivalent smokers. However, for some, once on the dependency treadmill it is very difficult to get off. Exactly how many smokers are addicted to nicotine is difficult to estimate. It probably ranges between 20 to 30 per cent of all smokers, which rates nicotine one of the most addictive substances known to man.

Not many non-smokers have much sympathy for addicted smokers, and smokers themselves are confused because they may have little objective understanding about what is going on with their own smoking and why they can't stop it.

We know that there is nothing 'mentally' wrong with these smokers. There is no evidence that they have any personality disorders. Many psychological tests have been carried out to see whether smokers who are addicted to nicotine have something in common with each other, and are therefore different from the smokers that have quit and from non-smokers. There seems to be no parameter tested so far that picks an addicted smoker out of the crowd, except, ironically, their lack of self-efficacy in quitting. That is, they doubt their own ability to quit. Neither age, sex nor years of smoking influence the addiction. No social barrier exists either. Addicts come from all walks of life, from judges to cleaners, doctors and factory workers. We also know that addicted smokers are fully aware of the medical implications of what they are doing. It is not from lack of information about the adverse effects of smoking that stops these smokers from quitting.

What is most intriguing, frustrating and annoying is that there are some smokers who apparently quit smoking effortlessly, the ambivalent smoker who can take it or leave it, while other smokers find doing this a hopelessly distressing event. This is not unlike drinking and alcoholism. Most people drink alcohol and show no dependency at all to it, however, some do get addicted and they find it extremely difficult to stop drinking. This is not due to an attitude to the substance in question. It is the individual's biological reaction to the chemical—nicotine or alcohol—that is different. Why does one person have this reaction and not the other and why one chemical and not the other? There is mounting evidence that an individual's reaction to nicotine may be inherited, and that even difficulty in quitting may be inherited. It is in the neurons, the brain cells, that the addicted smoker will be picked out from the crowd. The brain's reaction to nicotine is different in each individual and this leads to the varying reactions and degrees of addiction that people have and the difficulties they experience when they try to stop using it.

What is an addiction?

The World Health Organisation (WHO) defines an addiction or dependency using three main criteria:

1. That a substance is used on a regular basis to maintain a blood level, to which a tolerance develops.
2. That the substance is used to prevent withdrawals and causes relapse.
3. That the substance is used in the face of known physical and social detriment.

How does this apply to smoking?

Nicotine

It needs to be made clear that it is the nicotine and no other chemical in cigarettes that makes people smoke. Without nicotine there is little interest in smoking as there is no other chemical in tobacco that has any psychopharmacological effect. You don't see rows and rows of herbal cigarettes in the duty-free stores or in the supermarkets. They are not big sellers because the vital ingredient of nicotine is missing.

So for a better understanding of the problem of smoking it is important to know more about the chemistry of nicotine, as it has such a profound effect on why and how it is used.

Nicotine comes from the tobacco plant and cannot be made synthetically in a laboratory. The topmost leaves of the plant have the higher concentrations of nicotine and the bottom larger leaves and stalk have less. Combining different parts of the plant and different tobacco strains in the factory gives different concentrations of the chemical and thus different brands. Nicotine is an odourless, colourless alkaloid and is best absorbed in an alkaline environment, not an acidic environment. For example, smokers prefer to smoke with an alkaline such as coffee or alcohol where the absorption through the mouth is better than, say, with a citrus fruit juice which is acidic and makes the absorption of nicotine too slow.

It is interesting to note that the use of tobacco in Australia did not originate with European settlers. Australian Aborigines had long been using the tobacco plant *Nicotiana hopwoodii*, called *pituri*, for thousands of years. Pharmaco-anthropologist Pamela Watson from the University of Queensland discovered that the

NICOTINE IS NOT STORED IN THE BODY; IT LASTS 12 HOURS.

Aborigines had used the power of the nicotine plant to kill animals, and certain elders chewed the plant themselves. It was considered a prize possession and was bartered for all over Australia. *Pituri* still grows wild in northern Queensland.

Today nicotine use is widespread and through trial and error the way nicotine gets into the blood and then to the brain has been optimised and has become very sophisticated. Man has refined ways of getting the chemical quickly into the brain. Chewing it, sniffing it and inhaling it seem to get the best results. Eating it, that is ingestion, has never been popular because nicotine is almost completely neutralised in the acids of the stomach, where little absorption takes place. However, it travels from the lungs through to the brain in about seven seconds, so that inhaling it is about the quickest way to get the required amount of nicotine. Injecting nicotine into the arm could not get it to the brain as fast as inhaling it does. The speed with which this drug enters the brain is the main reason that it has become so addictive.

Described below are each of the main criterion of addiction, as they pertain to tobacco use.

Maintaining a nicotine blood level

Part one of the WHO definition of an addiction states maintaining a blood level of a drug is critical.

The main reason behind the need to smoke again once nicotine is in the blood is because the half-life of nicotine is very short—from about 40 to 100 minutes. This means that about 40 minutes after having a cigarette the nicotine from it is reduced to half its strength. The whole-life of nicotine is much longer, about twelve hours. So after twelve hours all the nicotine in the bloodstream has been worn down, or metabolised, and there is very little left. There is no long-term storage of nicotine anywhere in the body. This is why so many addicted smokers need to smoke first thing in the morning. Their nicotine blood level is extremely low and they find it very difficult to get going without it.

Nicotine is metabolised or broken up by the liver and kidneys. Its main breakdown substance is called cotinine, which is found in the bloodstream up to two days after a cigarette is smoked. Cotinine has no pharmacological activity in the body and is mainly urinated out but is also excreted in saliva. Nicotine can be detected inside the hair of smokers, is found in breast milk and passes freely through the placenta into the amniotic fluid in pregnancy.

Exactly what the blood level of nicotine is in each smoker varies. A major error made by most smokers is that they assume the amount of nicotine they get from a cigarette is the amount described on the packet. For example, a 1.2 mg nicotine cigarette does not deliver 1.2 mg nicotine into the bloodstream. If it did there would be an immediate toxic reaction and very high levels of nicotine can be fatal. The concentration received from a cigarette is diluted a thousandfold. Nonetheless, most smokers know when their blood levels are too low or too high. They have a remarkable sensitivity to even the slightest variation in concentration cigarettes can deliver. The fact that for some a cigarette tastes strong or weak merely indicates that the amount of nicotine that cigarette is delivering is not right for them.

Experiments have been carried out where the amount of nicotine in cigarettes has been changed without smokers being aware. If the cigarette was low they immediately began to smoke differently, inhaling deeper and complaining of the taste. If the cigarette was higher in nicotine content they would puff lightly without inhaling deeply.

Filters have changed the manner of smoking quite dramatically, as have low-nicotine cigarettes. With the advent of these, the amount of nicotine delivered to the smoker became lower. To compensate, a smoker often either draws back harder on the cigarette or smokes more of them to achieve the required blood level. For example, many smokers have gone over to lower nicotine-content cigarettes in the hope that they are somehow better for their health. Unfortunately they may have to inhale deeper on the cigarette or smoke more cigarettes to compensate for the low nicotine levels. It is no coincidence that today there are few cigarette packets that have twenty in them; most have at least twenty-five. The lower the nicotine, the more in the box. There are even very low nicotine cigarettes with 50 in the box! Either way, by using a filter or smoking lower concentrations, the nicotine in the blood remains basically the same as it always was. More evidence that it is the nicotine in the cigarette that controls the smoking.

Nicotine in the brain

Neurotransmitters are chemicals that help pass electrical impulses from one brain cell or neuron to the other. There are many neurotransmitters in the body. The best known neurotransmitter is adrenaline, but other well-known neurotransmitters are the endorphins— acetylcholine, and dopamine. It is suspected that there are many thousands yet undiscovered and that each has its own specific function and site at which it works. Some function only in the brain; their job may be to relieve pain, others are for relaxation. Some only work in the body to induce muscle contraction, others for muscle relaxation. We know that nicotine acts actively in the brain as a neurotransmitter substance. This means that it enhances activity in the brain cells, allowing electrical impulses to pass from one cell to the next.

It is believed that nicotine is in fact a very good neurotransmitter and is very efficient at doing this. Smokers develop nicotine receptor sites to take up nicotine in their neurons. Certain areas of the brain are more affected by this than others. For example, research has shown that smokers do not see or hear any better with or without a cigarette, but with the use of nicotine they may be able to remember things better and perform tasks that require concentration better when they have nicotine bathing their brain cells than when they don't. This of course does not mean that non-smokers can't do these things! It means that with this substance continually in the brain smokers have become 'lazy' and don't use their own neurotransmitters. Electroencephalograms, EEGs, measure electrical activity in the brain. The EEG changes from fast to slow waves when a smoker is deprived of nicotine.

It becomes understandable then that when a smoker is attempting to quit, eliminating nicotine altogether, the brain cells find this very distressing. Imagine if there was something wrong with your kidneys. You usually get an indication that things are not well: you may get pain and pass bloody urine. In the case of the smoker, when the brain is deprived of nicotine it expresses its unwellness often with behavioural changes. You may well say 'my brain hurts'. These are the gamut of withdrawals that are described below as the Nicotine Withdrawal Syndrome, which is now well recognised to occur in many smokers trying not to smoke, and fit the WHO criteria for dependency.

The strangest chemical effect of nicotine is that it can have two opposing reactions, depending on the dose. If a high dose of nicotine is extracted from a cigarette it can have a calming effect, and if low doses are extracted it can have a stimulating effect. Some smokers may know that when they are excited and rushed, a long drag on a cigarette will slow them down and conversely when they are bored and lethargic a few quick puffs will pick them up.

Tolerance

In pharmacological terms tolerance is akin to its other meanings in English. It simply means that when a chemical initially has a reaction in a person it will often diminish with continued use until, sometimes, there is no reaction at all. The person then tolerates the drug. If however you are seeking a reaction, as in say drinking alcohol, you will need more and more alcohol to elicit an effect. Some drinkers can drink a lot without too much of an effect; others who don't drink often are knocked around by even a little alcohol. They have no tolerance to it. Eventually big drinkers need to drink more and more to achieve the desired effect. This also occurs in smoking, but in a strange manner. Unlike drinking, the amount of cigarettes doesn't increase over the years. It may in the very beginning, but eventually most smokers achieve a standard amount they use and this remains stable for years and years. This is because tolerance to nicotine dissipates very quickly, sometimes even between cigarettes. A good example of this happens to many smokers. If the early morning cigarette is delayed for any reason, or it has been many hours since the last cigarette, when a cigarette is finally smoked the smoker can be quite affected. They may have an increased heart rate, and feel dizzy and nauseous. They have lost their tolerance to it. But with the next cigarette this effect is gone, and the tolerance has been re-established.

Nicotine and other chemicals
Alcohol
Nicotine and alcohol interreact powerfully in the brain. They have what is called a synergynistic effect, that is, 1+1=3. They enhance each other and increase the need for each other. The effect is so profound that most smokers, of all types, will increase their intake of cigarettes to at least double while they are drinking. In the time span they have a drink, many increase by three or four times the amount they would normally smoke. Most smokers believe that the social effect of drinking is the main cause for the increase, and that alcohol reduces your inhibitions. This is true. However, we also know that alcohol affects the neurons that are sensitive to nicotine and heightens their reactions. You only have

to look at a smoker who drinks. Even without friends around or without being in the club or pub, just drinking alone will increase the need to smoke. With these reactions occurring, it is little wonder that smokers find it almost impossible to drink and not smoke.

Caffeine

The interaction between nicotine and caffeine is not the same as with alcohol. There is no enhancement of the need to smoke with caffeine intake per se, but lately some startling evidence has shown that nicotine reduces blood levels of caffeine (not the other way around). Simply put, this means most smokers are going to need to have two cups of coffee for one that a non-smoker has. Some smokers, though, have made strong associations with coffee and a cigarette break. This may happen because the coffee, or tea for that matter, is the legitimate break they have to be able to smoke. The association is part of the breaking away from an activity, a stop–think pause in the day. (Caffeine use has not been demonstrated as addictive. Animals will not self-administer caffeine.)

Marijuana

This drug, often smoked along with tobacco, seems to have an influence on the need to smoke cigarettes. Many cigarette smokers smoke marijuana. Whereas it would be very strange for a non-smoker to light up a joint, it is not foreign for a smoker to smoke per se, so they are more likely to smoke something else. The mechanism by which marijuana enhances the need to smoke is not known but it is certain that marijuana smoking can cause the need to smoke cigarettes and possibly vice versa. Smoking marijuana has often been cited as the cause of young people taking up smoking cigarettes, but studies have also shown that it is common for many young smokers of cigarettes to move from tobacco to marijuana and then on to other illicit drugs.

Other drugs and nicotine
Most illicit drug users smoke. When we studied smoking in heroin addicts attending a methadone unit we noted that 98 per cent were smokers, and most showed a very high physical addiction to tobacco. When we asked them confidentially which drug they preferred to stop using they said they would rather stop doing any other drug rather than have to stop smoking. They rated tobacco as giving them the severest withdrawals of all.

The nicotine withdrawal syndrome

Again, according to the criteria of addictions, withdrawals from the substance used needs to occur to be able to claim that an addiction is present. The nicotine withdrawal syndrome has been well documented in many medical journals and has recently been entered into a massive psychiatric medical text, *The Diagnostic and Statistical Manual of the American Psychiatric Association* (the *DSM*), the bible of psychiatrists.

Because the very nature of the withdrawals affect behaviour many smokers and some therapists erroneously believe that smoking has masked or suppressed an emotional state that really exists within them, and that when they attempt to quit this new personality is exposed. Withdrawals such as anxiety, irritability and aggression add weight to their beliefs. However, withdrawals are transient events that dissipate in time, and are not due to inherent personality traits.

The withdrawals listed below do not occur in everyone and not all of them occur. Some people less addicted may have none of them, but some more addicted may unfortunately have them all.

Within hours of not smoking:

Cravings
Anxiety
Irritability
Lack of concentration
Nervousness
Tension

Within 24 hours of not smoking:

Hypersomnia/insomnia
Headaches
Cramps
Light-headedness
Constipation
Increase in appetite, especially for sweet foods

Some longer-term symptoms after many days of not smoking:

Memory loss
Mouth ulcers
Cough
Grief
Depression
Curiosity about using tobacco again

Relapse

Relapsing is epidemic amongst smokers. It is estimated that between 70 and 80 per cent of all smokers have made at least one attempt to quit smoking unsuccessfully. Ninety-five per cent of smokers who have a lapse, that is even a single cigarette, relapse to full-on smoking. Some researchers believe that smokers even relapse between cigarettes; others feel that only after

24 hours of abstinence does smoking again constitute a relapse. Whichever the definition, it is certain that it is the withdrawals listed above that drive most smokers to doing it again. Another part of the problem of relapse is due to the learning experienced by smokers.

The learning process of smoking

Having described how the basis for continuous smoking is the maintenance of a steady flow of nicotine into the brain, it is equally important to understand how this then becomes the ingrained behaviour that some smokers call the psychological component of smoking or the 'bad habit' part. There is no real need to separate the physiological and psychological need to smoke. The principle is the same, for example, as eating. Basically the body needs nutrients to survive. The way the body says 'top me up' is to have your stomach rumble. You get hungry and so you eat. Then you learn to eat regularly so as not to run out of nutrients. First the physiology, then the psychology—both interwoven.

The reactions with smoking are somewhat the same. You run out of nicotine very quickly; this makes you anxious so you learn to 'top up' so as not to run out. This then becomes an ingrained reaction that lasts for years and sometimes decades. Fortunately the body can survive without nicotine, but it cannot survive without food.

The other learning component is what psychologists call 'positive reinforcement'. When you are hungry, you eat and then you feel good; when you get anxious and you smoke, you feel good. These are two examples of positive reinforcement. The effects are also instantaneous, particularly in smoking. A smoker can feel down, upset and irritable, smoke a cigarette and immediately feel better. Every smoker knows that the chemical effect is instant. Nicotine is a powerful positive reinforcer.

A VICIOUS CIRCLE

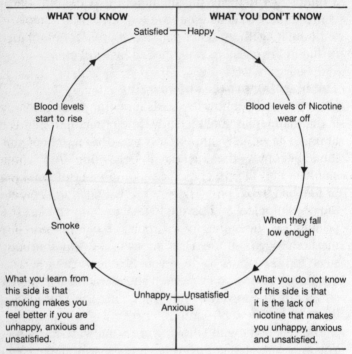

WHAT YOU KNOW	WHAT YOU DON'T KNOW

Satisfied — Happy

Blood levels start to rise

Blood levels of Nicotine wear off

Smoke

When they fall low enough

What you learn from this side is that smoking makes you feel better if you are unhappy, anxious and unsatisfied.

Unhappy — Unsatisfied
Anxious

What you do not know of this side is that it is the lack of nicotine that makes you unhappy, anxious and unsatisfied.

Once you have learned the left-side it is instilled in your brain even when you do not smoke any longer. You will, however, gradually un-learn this.

What the smoker has learned from all of this is 'smoking makes me feel better'. What the smoker does not know and has not learned is that it is the withdrawals from nicotine that often make you feel bad in the first place.

The learning experience is also known as conditioning or, more specifically, Pavlovian conditioning. This conditioning is the primary problem in relapsing.

Smoking in the face of knowing it's bad for you

This is remarkably common. In fact almost every smoker

today knows at least some of the detrimental effects of smoking. It is written blatantly on the packet of every box of cigarettes and can hardly be ignored. But part of the WHO definition of addiction is that you use the substance in the face of the social and medical implications. We know that some people with heart, lung or vascular disease go on smoking despite dire warnings from their doctors. We have had cases of patients lying to their surgeons to be able to have their operations, asthmatics in severe distress still smoking and patients smoking through the holes in their tracheas after tracheotomies. They do not do this out of defiance or ignorance but out of dependency and because addictions override all rationalisation.

Today we know that one in three pregnant women smoke. One would imagine that these women would be strongly influenced to quit 'for the sake of the baby'. Many would be able to stop if they were pointed in the right direction, but many are simply addicted. There is also undoubted social pressure to quit. The anti-smoking climate has made smoking extremely uncomfortable for many smokers. No smoking in public venues, theatres, restaurants, transport, the workplace and many private homes has pushed some smokers literally into the closet. They feel themselves social pariahs. To some it has become a huge embarrassment, to others an aggression on their civil liberties which they defy having imposed on them. Whichever the reaction, the smoker often has to negotiate a place to go to be able to smoke. The true nature of an addiction becomes apparent when you have to go find yourself a spot, any spot, where you can have a cigarette.

Imagine now a day in the life of a typically addicted smoker. It becomes more understandable:

On waking up in the morning after an eight-hour sleep,

there is little nicotine left in the bloodstream. The kidneys and the liver have broken much of it down, metabolised it, and the remnants are in the bladder where it is urinated out. There is no store of it anywhere in the body. The brain, now awake, is like any machine that is turned on: it needs oil in the motor—the red light is flashing. So the first cigarette of the day is usually smoked within five to twenty minutes of waking. The level of nicotine rises sharply in the brain. Sometimes two cigarettes need to be smoked to achieve the required dose. The addicted smoker can now function normally. Unfortunately, the level drops pretty quickly soon after and within half an hour the level is about half of what it was. This precipitous drop is striking and the smoker will need to have another cigarette to stop the level falling to what it was on waking.

NO PRODUCTS FROM SMOKING COME OUT OF THE PORES OF YOUR SKIN.

The whole day is spent 'topping up' to keep the level from falling too low. There is a slow accumulated rise of the baseline of nicotine over the day so some smokers will find that they may smoke more in the earlier part of the day than the later part. A typical reaction to the drop in nicotine blood levels over six hours is shown below. As the blood levels drop, the smoker is thinking more and more about a cigarette.

The blood levels of nicotine in the graph are in nanograms (ng). A nanogram is one thousandth of a gram (g) or a hundredth of a milligram (mg). This means that by the time a cigarette of say 1.2 mg is smoked the actual amount entering the blood is diluted extensively.

Unlike other drugs of addiction, nicotine does not give an 'out of body experience' or a 'high'. It primarily maintains normality. This means that when it wears off

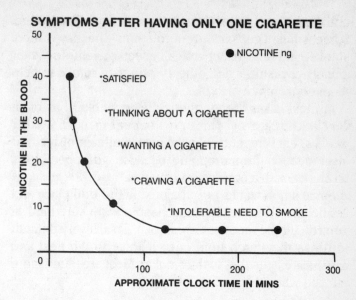

SYMPTOMS AFTER HAVING ONLY ONE CIGARETTE

NICOTINE ng

*SATISFIED

*THINKING ABOUT A CIGARETTE

*WANTING A CIGARETTE

*CRAVING A CIGARETTE

*INTOLERABLE NEED TO SMOKE

NICOTINE IN THE BLOOD

APPROXIMATE CLOCK TIME IN MINS

the smoker will get anxious and nervous and when they smoke again they will feel calm and relaxed, i.e. normal. It is not that smokers are by nature nervous people, it is that the withdrawals make them very nervous, even between cigarettes. A smoker is usually satisfied after a cigarette but in about two hours there is a serious need to smoke again. Most addicts would find four hours to be the maximum time they can hold out. Some smoke right until going to bed. It is believed that during the night the brain, though still active, doesn't need nicotine for these activities, so the smoker doesn't wake to have a cigarette. However, if they do wake up for any other reason, some smokers then, because they have become mobilised and active, need a cigarette as if it was first thing in the morning.

However, not all smokers are addicted to the same degree so that the description of one smoker may be unlike another smoker whose dependency is less severe. Some smoke consistently throughout the day, others smoke only for the chemical effect of relieving their anxiety or distress, and others again may smoke to help them concentrate on a task.

In most cases though the addicted smoker has often very little control over his or her behaviour. Each waking day is spent very much like the next, maintaining a blood level to stop it from dropping, because a dropped blood level means discomfort and cravings.

Since smoking has been banned in the workplace and is socially undesirable some people work very hard at controlling the amount they smoke. This is very difficult to do as they lurch from one cigarette to the next and causes great distress to the smoker. Most are much more relaxed when they can smoke liberally.

Women and smoking

There have been long, heated debates over whether women have a bigger problem with smoking than men, and whether they should be catered for in a category of their own. There are certainly more women smoking in our society than men. Why they have taken up smoking in such vast numbers is a complex combination of the financial liberation of women in our society, coupled with specific image advertising targeted at women which then leads on to formidable peer-group pressure. Whether women have a more difficult time in quitting smoking is altogether different from whether more women smoke than men. There is little evidence to prove that withdrawals are worse, or that relapse rates are more severe in women. Even that perpetual problem that plagues women today, that of weight gain, seems not to be a reason for women to relapse. In other words gaining weight is not a cause of relapse in women who quit, but the *fear* of gaining weight may be the major reason women do not even attempt to quit. Thus women per se are not more addicted to nicotine than men.

Animal models

Animal models give us an insight into the usage of drugs that are unclouded by complex human behaviours.

It is relatively easy to get other animals besides humans to self-administer nicotine. But they do not do this by learning to smoke. In fact it is extremely difficult to teach any animal to smoke. The self-administration comes in the form of a shot of nicotine through an intravenous drip that the animal can trigger through pressing on a lever. A great deal of information has been gained through these types of animal experiments. Most of the animals used are rats and, like humans, certain strains of rats are more likely to become dependent on nicotine than others. Their reactions to nicotine are remarkably similar to humans. They get symptoms of withdrawal, become tolerant to the adverse chemical effects, and persist in self-administration in the face of adversity.

Tests done with rats have been extremely helpful in learning about addictions. For example, rats can be given difficult tasks to carry out and are rewarded with a dose of nicotine. As the tasks become more and more difficult they will not give up trying until it becomes extraordinarily difficult to achieve a reward. These results have been interpreted by some to mean that if the cost, either financial or health-wise, becomes great, addicts will not give up unless the costs are extraordinarily high. The evidence in human behaviour regarding cigarette smoking confirms this. Often neither extreme ill health nor large price rises restrain smokers. Other experiments have shown that the environment in which the animal becomes dependent, that is, a particular cage, will become the place the animal experiences withdrawals and seeks the drug. If they recover from withdrawals somewhere else, they will get them again when placed back in the original environment. If they experience the withdrawals in the original environment they will recover well. This has an implication on humans as well in how and where they attempt to quit.

In summary nicotine is a powerful pharmacological agent. Now that a great deal more is known about it and its addictive properties it is appropriate to move on to assessing it in an individual smoker doing something about its use.

☺ 2 ☺

Self-assessment

It is evident from the previous chapter that there are varying degrees of dependency on nicotine just as there are in any other drug dependencies. If we know how severe the addiction is, we can find better ways of combating it.

Here are four examples of people who all smoke and who all find it difficult to quit. They are not different by their type of addiction but by the severity of it, some having it mildly and others having it severely.

Mary has made lots of attempts to quit smoking and has succeeded often for three to four weeks, and for some of the time when she was pregnant. However, when something dramatic happens, she fights with her friend or she gets a huge telephone bill, she'll decide to just have one to calm her down. Immediately Mary's back to smoking again. She smokes with a drink at night, but during the day she has little need to smoke—maybe having one if the kids get on her nerves or as a treat after doing some chore. She'll sit down and relax with her friend the cigarette. She wouldn't dream of smoking at her parents' place or in the car. Mary's cravings for cigarettes occur with certain occasions or activities, and with alcohol.

Bill starts the day off in bed with a cigarette or two to get him going. He often skips breakfast and takes off to work smoking in the car on the way. He has great difficulty not smoking at work since it's been banned there, and he often has to duck out to have a cigarette on the fire stairs. On the weekends he smokes as much as during the week. He's tried to stop and knows he should but he has never really had a day without smoking because the cravings get too tough and he gets so agitated that he can't concentrate at work.

Jan has been smoking for forty years. She lives alone and cigarettes are her best friend. Jan is unaware that she smokes routinely throughout the day at set times; she does it automatically. The cigarettes keep her company, she knows that much. She keeps reiterating that smoking 'isn't doing her any good' but since her doctor told her that she has chronic bronchitis she feels it's too late to stop anyway, and after all, it would be too difficult at her age having smoked all these years. Jan also gets a little depressed and takes some sleeping tablets to help her sleep at night. What really bothers her are her grandchildren complaining that 'Nana stinks' and she'd like to do something about it for them, but altogether she isn't very motivated to quit because she doesn't believe she can.

Stan is a businessman, has had two heart attacks and has had bypass surgery. He smokes fifteen a day, and tries very hard not to smoke every one of them. Stan lies to the cardiologist who takes care of him about his smoking. Stan is afraid that the cardiologist would refuse to treat him. Stan wakes up every morning wanting not to smoke. He sincerely wishes that the cravings wouldn't overwhelm him and he is fully aware of the impact smoking has on his heart, but Stan does it anyway. Stan has a serious mental conflict. His wife is very concerned about his health and is constantly at him. He's always finding excuses to get out of the house, buy a paper, walk the dog etc. Ironically all this makes Stan more nervous and he smokes more when he is thinking whether he should smoke or not!

All four have tried to quit and can't. Some people smoke so infrequently that it hardly seems worth it. How is it that Mary smokes mostly at night with a drink when Bill can't get out of bed without a cigarette and smokes full-on all day? You would also assume that Stan, who is highly motivated and has a desperate need to quit, should be able to do so, whereas Jan, who is less

---

DRINKING A LOT OF WATER WILL NOT FLUSH YOUR SYSTEM OF TOXINS FROM SMOKING.

---

motivated, would find it very difficult. Each has reacted differently to the effects of nicotine.

These reactions are likened to an allergy. If you are allergic to, say, tomatoes, you may get a small pimply rash on your arm or get a rash on your chest and face or you may even break out in huge welts all over your body. The reaction varies in each individual. Of course most people have no reaction to tomatoes at all and can eat them without any side effects. The variation is not in the psychological make up of the person but more in the body chemistry. Smokers react similarly to nicotine. Some manifest huge dependencies, others very weak ones and some have none at all. There is also no relationship to the length of time you have been smoking. That is, you would expect that the addiction gets worse over the years but that does not seem to be the case.

Just like an allergy to tomatoes it crosses all age, sex and social backgrounds and how long you've been exposed. All this is the reason why some people have no trouble quitting. (*They give 'giving up' a good name!!!*) And some have such terrible trouble. Stan is using cigarettes in the face of what he knows is bad for him. There is no doubt that most smokers are aware of the ill effects of smoking, but only truly addicted smokers will persist in smoking if they get sick themselves. It is not unusual for smokers with emphysema and other severe respiratory diseases to go on smoking. There's no such thing as 'too sick to smoke'. In some people that includes being in hospital.

In the past we thought smoking was primarily a bad habit that had mostly to do with emotional states, so old questionnaires have asked details about being bored or feelings that might be negative or positive when you started to think about smoking. We also used to ask about handling a cigarette. Today we have advanced from these questions and have been able to get a better detail of the level of physical dependency by asking other sorts of questions relating to the topography, or technique, of smoking.

The Dependency Questionnaire

The Fagerström Dependency Questionnaire was devised by Karl-Olov Fagerström, a Swede, who developed these questions so that a better diagnosis could be made of each smoker. Fagerstrom found that there was a correlation between the score reached and symptoms of withdrawal. He found that the higher you scored, the worse the withdrawals would likely be and the harder it would be for you to quit smoking unaided.

Once you can better define how dependent you are

you can better gear yourself to a course of action to stop smoking. It sounds self-evident, that you have a good notion of your own dependency, however this is rarely true. Most smokers have never been able to assess themselves in this objective manner before. This of course is not a foolproof questionnaire as some smokers, even though they may score a low level in dependency, still find it difficult to quit as the physical withdrawals are not that severe but the social pull to smoke is very strong. This is often due to social conditioning where you have learned to smoke in a particular situation but outside of that the urge to smoke is not there.

You have to be absolutely honest with yourself when you answer the questions. There is nobody looking over your shoulder when you score yourself. If you truly do

> TAKING VITAMIN C WILL NOT HELP YOU STOP SMOKING.

not know the answer to some questions then wait a day and pay strict attention to what you are doing on that day. For example, you may truly not know how many cigarettes a day you smoke because you never keep count, or you have no idea whether it's worse in the morning than the evening. You may also have packets lying everywhere so you can't keep track. Take a day to pay attention to it. Each lit cigarette counts. Don't count half a cigarette smoked as half a cigarette because it counts as a whole one!

Pipe and cigar smokers

Though many pipe and cigar smokers feel they are better off physically with this sort of smoking, they may not be aware of the dependency being as severe as in any other type of smoking. Pipe and cigar smokers have exactly the same problems quitting as cigarette smokers. It is no easier.

It is very common for cigarette smokers who have gone over to smoking cigars to smoke them as if they were cigarettes, lighting them frequently and inhaling deeply. For a self-assessment in cigar and pipe smokers, you should count every time you light or relight the cigar or pipe as if it were a single cigarette smoked. The nicotine content will always be the highest even though it is not mentioned on the packaging. It needs to be stressed that they are regular, i.e. daily smokers of pipes or cigars who find it difficult not to smoke every day and not the person who smokes the odd cigar infrequently.

You may also believe that you never inhale from your cigarette. This is extremely rare. If you do not do this often that is different from never doing it.

You will notice that there is no mention of the social situations around your smoking. Most smokers feel that where they are and what they are doing is very important to their smoking. Also that handling and lighting a cigarette, watching the smoke rise from the ashtray etc., has an impact on their actual need to smoke. These are strong triggers and cues and are very important in staying stopped, but there seems to be no evidence that they have an effect on the physical aspect of smoking.

		Points
How soon after you wake do you smoke your first cigarette?	within 30 min	0
	after 30 min	1
Do you find it difficult to refrain from smoking in places where it is forbidden, e.g. at meetings,		

		Points
at the library, in cinemas etc.?	yes	1
	no	0
Which cigarette would you hate to give up?	The first one in the morning	1
	any other	0
How many cigarettes a day do you smoke?	15 or less	0
	16–25	1
	26 or more	2
Do you smoke more frequently during the morning than during the rest of the day?	yes	1
	no	0
Do you smoke if you are so ill that you are in bed most of the day?	yes	1
	no	0
What is the nicotine level of your usual brand of cigarettes? (Check the pack for this information.)	0.9 mg or less	0
	1.0–1.2 mg	1
	1.3 mg or more	2
Do you inhale?	never	0
	sometimes	1
	always	2

How to tally up the scores:
The maximum score is eleven. Fagerström has divided the scores up so that if you score between 1–5 you are mildly dependent; if you score from 6–7 you are moderately dependent; and if you score from 8–11 you show severe dependency.

CATEGORY	A	B	C
	Score 0–5	Score 6–7	Score 8–11

These categories are explored in greater detail in chapter 3.

In the above test someone like Mary would score between 1–5, while Jan would score a 7 and Bill and Stan would score 8 plus.

Another judgment of dependency is based on how long you can go without a cigarette. At our clinic we ask every smoker how long is the longest they went without smoking *at all* in their whole smoking career. The average we found was one month, but it ranged from a few hours to several days. If you have only been able to not smoke for a maximum of several days then we would also consider you to be severely dependent. If it has been several weeks to a month then you are moderately dependent. If you have been able to remain abstinent more than once for up to three months or more then we would class you as mildly dependent.

Two other major aspects some people believe influence their ability to quit are stress and depression.

Stress

Many people confuse stress with being busy. Many of us lead very busy lives, with problems that need to be solved immediately, deadlines that have to be met or difficult people that have to be dealt with. If we know that one of the side effects of the wearing off of nicotine is anxiety and that re-administering nicotine helps it go away, then we know that someone with a busy lifestyle is going to deal with individual stressful moments with a cigarette because they will feel much better and less distressed doing so. Having learned to do this and received the positive effects from this every time, a 'stressed' smoker has what they believe to be a great disadvantage in trying to quit. Though certain incidents are triggers, a stressful or busy life is not considered to be contrary to quitting smoking and should not pose any major problem. It certainly should not be used as a reason not to quit. What can be done about the stressful triggers is described in the next chapters.

Depression

Unlike stress, any medical history of depression does have an effect on the ability to quit smoking. If there has been a need to take anti-depressants in the past, a smoker like this should grade themselves up one category to B if they scored an A, or to C if they scored B.

⊘ 3 ⊘

How to stop doing it

This chapter presents different ways to actually stop
smoking. That is, not putting cigarettes into your mouth
any more. This is different from keeping it that way, or
maintaining abstinence, which is a separate issue and
is dealt with further on in this book. Using the same
example of the allergy, this section deals with treating
the rash you got from eating tomatos and deals with
teaching you to stay away from them.

All smokers, however, have the same initial problem.
'Do I really want to do this?' When it comes to the crunch,
the decision to stop smoking for life, to stop doing
something that you've been doing for years on end, is
a really daunting one. Secretly smokers may think: *Is
there life without smoking?*' 'How can I possibly answer
the phone or drink a glass of beer without a cigarette?'
'I really like it.' When it all boils down to it, it seems
that the decision to actually do something about your
smoking is a question of *maturity*. This doesn't mean
age. When you were young you were told 'you're not
old enough to smoke,' but now you may well ask yourself,
'Am I old enough to *not* smoke?' 'Do I really want to
put this behind me?'

Now that you know more about the chemical nicotine

and its involvement in your smoking, your attitude towards your smoking may have changed quite considerably. You may now have become aware just how drug dependent you are. The fact that it is not an arbitrary bad habit but may be a behaviour over which you've had little control may make you wish to take some control over it now. No rational person wants a drug dictating their behaviour. You may never have realised that it is not 'all in the mind' but more 'all in the brain'.

Every day there is some revolutionary new method that is supposed to be the only way that smokers can quit. (There are some smokers having read this book so far nodding their heads.) They've seen and heard it all before. The most unfortunate part of these experiences is that smokers invest time and money on these methods and are very disappointed when they don't help. So much so that any future attempts to quit are put off because they consider themselves hopeless cases. This in itself is why some methods are so counterproductive . . . those who need help most don't get it and are put off forever.

Smokers who are in the addicted category often resort to outside help to quit. They may have attempted to quit on many occasions on their own and found it too difficult, gone off to a chemist and bought what they thought might be the 'magic bullet'. There have been millions of dollars made on this magic bullet without much benefit to the consumer. Many unsubstantiated claims of 80 to 90 per cent success in quitting are made for a variety a lotions, potions and courses on the market, none of which have ever been properly assessed or had any scientific evaluation. When they have been evaluated they simply do not pass the test.

What however can we say about the person who does quit using some quaint potion for which they paid an inordinate amount of money? The ability to quit was probably due to what is called the 'placebo effect'. Simply taking something, anything, and paying for it (the more you pay the stronger the effect) has a psychological impact. It is as if the investment itself is enough of an incentive to push you along. Interestingly too, the more invasive the therapy, the stronger the placebo effect. For example, a pill is less effective than a needle, which is less effective than an intravenous drip, even if there is nothing in any of them. This is not to dismiss the placebo effect out of hand. The effect can and is utilised in all forms of medicine and therapies, ancient and modern. However, an awareness that this exists is important in evaluating any type of treatment for yourself before you buy into it. There are many proven and

> EXERCISING WILL NOT COUNTERBALANCE THE EFFECTS OF SMOKING.

effective ways to stop smoking above and beyond the placebo effect.

Many addicted smokers cannot and should not expect a simplistic remedy to their smoking. How many smokers have attended hypnotherapy and quit, and how many have attended and smoked on the doorstep as they left the therapist's office? Why the difference between the two? One is less dependent than the other. Does expectation have an effect? Part of the placebo reaction is the expectancy of a cure. The stronger your desire for a cure the stronger the effect. But there are always enormous limitations to these psychological reactions. To date there is no understanding as to how they work.

In 1992 more than 1000 smokers, still smoking, in Sydney were asked what type of therapy they had used to try to help them quit smoking in the past. Their attempts were unsuccessful as they were still smoking. Many had tried more than one type of technique. The average was four different methods for each smoker.

Their choice was as follows:

	%
Cold turkey	64.3
Cutting down	52.6
Nicotine gum	43.1
Hypnotherapy	29.0
Acupuncture	19.2
Courses	10.6
'Other'	7.1
Herbal cures	5.9
Cigarette substitues	5.5
Lotions/creams	1.2

The list indicates just how often and how seriously smokers are taking their attempts to quit. They were choosing treatments they thought might help them, but it also indicates how singularly unsuccessful they were.

If you have measured your own level of dependency in the previous chapter you will be able to choose a method of quitting that will be better suited to your type, so that you are not randomly attempting something that sounds good in theory as the smokers did above. You will be less likely to waste your time, money and energy in a futile exercise that is doomed. Many of your friends may have been able to quit unaided or tried one type of treatment that was unsuccessful for you. The difference between you and them is not in your personality, it is in the method you used in *your* attempt to quit. However, finding a method that works for you is really the ultimate test and not that easy.

Whatever it is, we know that the smoother the transition from smoking to not smoking is, the more likely that it is going to remain that way. If stopping is awful and filled with drama, anxiety and distress, then the smoker will not stay a non-smoker for very long. If a smoker takes on the attitude 'I'll tough it out' through the trauma of quitting, that smoker will not do very well in the long run either. This means the nicer time you have quitting, the better. How could it be a 'nice time'? If the way you stop is chosen correctly, to suit you, the whole event shouldn't be too bad and you're much more likely to remain a non-smoker for good.

The guide for quitting set out below is for each separate category of smoker. However, there are some aspects of quitting that all smokers have in common. There are the dilemmas of where and when to quit.

Where
Try to stop smoking in the comfort of your normal daily life and environment. It sounds theoretically good to go away to quit smoking but in practice it is unusual for an addict to remain abstinent on re-entering their usual environment. Too many people have quit on holidays or at special resorts, even in hospital, but have relapsed the moment they got home. Not smoking should be learnt in your daily routine, not in a situation that is not normal. But if your environment is changing permanently then this is excellent timing to quit. For example, if you're moving house or going to a new job it is a good opportunity because your new environment can become a smoke-free zone from the start and you have little acclimatisation to contend with; it's a fait accompli.

It is fascinating in fact to look at the adaptation that smokers have made in certain areas. Take public transport for example. When the bans were introduced there was a general outcry from smokers, who believed they would find it impossible to cope with. Now most smokers can tolerate not smoking on a bus without the thought of smoking even entering their heads.

Another example, though not as widespread, is the *bedroom*. Some smokers would *never* smoke in their bedroom no matter what. Exactly why not isn't evident because they may smoke like chimneys in every other part of the house. The bedroom remains sacred, and the very idea of a cigarette doesn't even occur to them there.

When you stop smoking this same notion extends to the rest of your house and environment. Of course there are many smokers so dependent that they simply cannot get out of bed without a cigarette.

When

Is there a good time to quit? There are always excuses that this is a bad time and one can always keep on putting it off forever. However there are truly some bad times, where the odds are stacked against you from the start. In everyone's life there are dramas; highs and lows. If the background noise in your life is stable then it's as good a time to quit as ever, but if there is currently a *major* crisis in your life, then leave quitting till things settle down. A stressful life is not considered a major crisis! Many business people use this as an excuse not to make an attempt to stop smoking. 'My life is too hectic—I have a stressful life with deadlines to meet.' The timing for this person is okay but the motivation is poor; this person just doesn't want to quit.

Around exam time is bad timing and so is Christmas and New Year, though after both when life returns to normal it's a good way to commence a new year with a resolution.

For women, quitting when you are premenstrual is also bad timing, especially if you suffer from PMT. It can make symptoms of withdrawal much worse. Wait till it's over and then start.

The other dilemma common to all quitters is whether to tell others about what you are doing. In the past people have been advised to make bets, or announce it to all their friends or even buddy up with someone else. It is advisable *not* to tell everyone you know that you're quitting. Again, telling everyone may sound good in theory but in practice it causes anxiety. Even the kindest, most supportive person may bother you as they want to know how you're going on a regular, boring basis, and this can often grate on your nerves. The subject comes up much too often for your own good. A quiet support is the preferred option.

THE DAMAGE IS DONE—IT'S TOO LATE TO QUIT. IT IS NEVER TOO LATE TO QUIT NO MATTER HOW ADVANCED THE ILLNESS IS.

Buddying up with someone else also sounds good in theory. Friends can do well together, but if they go up together then they usually come down together. It's better to keep the issue to yourself.

It often occurs that those friends or colleagues (wives or husbands as well) who are at you about every single cigarette you smoke don't even notice when you're not smoking. They were down your throat every time you lit up! It may take months before they notice, so the best way to play this is like a game and wait and see how long it takes for this person who always nags you to notice you don't smoke.

Other smokers are usually not very sympathetic because you are leaving the ranks, and non-smokers don't sympathise at all because they can't understand what all the fuss is about. So it's better to keep mum on the whole thing and not make any statements at all. If however you can report in to, say, your local doctor, then you have an independent person who will always be encouraging.

Do you set the quit date? On your birthday, or perhaps the first of the month etc.? Again this has often been recommended as a technique to help you build up to the event. The best advice is to start straight away without too much haggling over a date. How unsuccessful this type of prearranged date can be is the typical reactions people have had to a price rise in their cigarettes. How many smokers have said to themselves 'When it gets to a dollar a packet, I'll quit,' then 'When it gets to three dollars a packet, I'll quit,' etc. etc.

There are some methods of quitting that have been universally accepted and well tested scientifically, and some that have not been.

Mouth sprays and lotions
There have been many brands of mouth washes that usually contain silver nitrate or acetate. When combined with nicotine this gives a foul taste to the smoker. Usually an addicted smoker will continue to smoke despite this taste, so that the effects are no real deterrent. It may help in newly smoking adolescents but getting them to use the spray is the main obstacle there.

Cutting down
Most smokers at some stage try to cut down on their smoking. Now it is better understood that a certain blood level needs to be maintained and that there is a level below which most addicted smokers find too difficult. This is why cutting down can be achieved to a degree, but cutting out completely is extremely difficult to some.

There is no point in cutting down, lurching from one cigarette to the next, if the ultimate aim of cutting out altogether cannot be achieved. Those people who cut down like this eventually find their smoking slowly creeps up. It is simply easier to smoke more than to smoke less.

The other effect of cutting down can be physically very harmful. When some smokers smoke less cigarettes, they inhale deeper from the ones they do have. Inhaling very deeply releases more carbon monoxide, which has a profound effect on the blood. The reactions to this carbon monoxide are explained in more detail in chapter 3. Smoking few cigarettes (five to ten per day) is not always what it seems. Nonetheless a program is set out at the end of this chapter for those who feel that this is the tactic best suited to them, as it is the least intimidating. The idea of slowly giving away each cigarette is more comforting than abruptly arresting smoking. However, it must be followed rigorously so as not to allow smoking to creep up again.

Changing brands

Changing brands usually means changing the nicotine level in the cigarette down to a weaker strength. The aim again is a weaning down approach. This is in theory a clever notion. If the nicotine concentrations are gradually reduced over a few weeks to almost negligible amounts then the smoker could conceivably come off nicotine altogether, and some do. Unfortunately many smokers often compensate for the drop in nicotine by smoking more cigarettes. If a smoker says they smoke a packet a day, it could mean anything. A packet of cigarettes today can contain anything from 20 to 50 cigarettes. These mega-packets contain cigarettes low in nicotine. The tobacco companies are aware that a smoker will compensate and need more cigarettes over a day.

Again the total effect is counterproductive as the smoker smokes more, either by inhaling deeper or smoking more cigarettes. The chemical effects are much worse than if they had never changed brands.

Hypnotherapy and acupuncture

The two methods of quitting which have been available for years in varying forms are hypnotherapy and acupuncture. They are either carried out in groups or on a one-to-one basis. In both these techniques, when well-conducted clinical trials have been carried out, these methods do not test very well. In drug addictions per se these two therapies are not considered valuable. They should not however be dismissed out of hand as valueless. They are both techniques that can engender a calming state in individuals. This can be very important in the withdrawal process. There may be some advantage for those in Category A. However, neither of these methods have helped those severely dependent on nicotine.

Group therapy

Joining groups to attempt to stop smoking has been a way for various smokers to buddy up with other smokers to quit. It has also been a way for some organisations to gain a great deal of profit from a large group of smokers all at once. The justification behind this is that there are so many smokers they cannot possibly be dealt with individually so this is the most cost-effective way. The fact that they are all dependent on nicotine in varying degrees and have varying difficulties is ignored. The group co-ordinators hope that some of the problems that some of the smokers encounter are covered, and hope that it covers most of the smokers in the group. Addicted smokers are rarely recognised, let alone catered for. The acid test for group therapy is very negative.

Groups like these often recommend behavioural changes with quirky tips like tying up your cigarettes so they are difficult to get out or deferring a smoke by drinking lots of water. Some of these tips help, but tips to help smokers quit abound and are not in themselves dangerous, though many are based on myth (see mythologies) and have no scientific basis whatsoever.

There have been attempts to establish Smokers Anonymous groups based on the same format as Alcoholics Anonymous. Unlike AA, SA has been singularly unsuccessful. Unfortunately this is mainly due to the difference in the drugs involved and the physical and social effects that are so different.

Aversive therapy

This may sound particularly drastic but is an age-old therapy used to change behaviour. Put simplistically, it is like teaching the child not to cross the road by giving them a smack; they soon learn not to. In the past if Johnny was caught smoking, Dad would take him down to the shed and overdose him on a cigar or several cigarettes until he got nauseous or sick. This was quite effective and Johnny usually didn't ever smoke again. Why doesn't this happen to adult smokers when they over-smoke? They have developed a tolerance to the negative effects of the smoking, and become immune as it were to it (see chapter 1). Thus aversive therapy has to be very intense to succeed in adults. This can be carried out, and is relatively successful in moderately dependent smokers, Category B, but the therapy should always be carried out under clinical supervision.

Nicotine replacements

In the past ten years or so the idea of using nicotine to fight the addiction to it has seemed very strange to many smokers. They feel that this is simply transferring the addiction to another form of the same drug. Other people less well informed believe that you should not have any crutch when you're giving up (this harps back to the notion that smokers have no willpower or backbone). But the nicotine replacement therapies have been an enormous bonus in helping those smokers with a strong dependency on nicotine. Without this form of therapy they would never have been able to quit. These therapies have also been well tested and scientifically evaluated.

Choosing a way to quit according to your type
Category A
Most smokers fall into this category. If you have found that you are in this category of mild nicotine dependency, this does not mean that your ability to quit is taken for granted and will be easy. The transition from being a smoker to being a non-smoker is mostly going to depend on your attitude and time passing, and not so much on the fact that withdrawals are going to overwhelm you. You would be better off quitting cold turkey. Your major goal is the first four days; don't look any further ahead than that. Remember this advice below covers the first few days only. Some smokers may be in this category and have gone weeks without smoking without any problems. Staying stopped is their main problem. If this is the case, then follow the instructions below and then go on to chapter 5. Here are some tips for you to help you quit:

☻ Start first thing in the morning. When you wake up you have little nicotine in your bloodstream and the aim is to keep it a nicotine-free day.

☻ *Eat breakfast!* Many smokers never do. Don't

confuse a need to eat with a need to smoke. Energy can be derived from a cigarette and it is known to reduce hunger pangs. Do not smoke instead of eating.

☺ *NO ALCOHOL*! Alcohol stimulates the need to smoke at least threefold. Therefore, no drinking alcohol for at least two weeks while you're quitting. This does not mean *low* alcohol drinks, it means *no* alcohol drinks.

☺ Keep away from other people's cigarette smoke. The nicotine you inhale will trigger off a desire to smoke. Seeing other people smoke may also be a cue. Do not intentionally go to places where people smoke to test yourself out.

☺ Accessability to cigarettes is important. If you don't have them just there in front of you, if it takes a little effort to get them then you're more likely to reconsider using them, so toss the cigarettes in the boot of the car or store them in the freezer (not the fridge), *but* don't get rid of them altogether at first because this may make you very nervous, and that is something you must avoid becoming.

☺ Tasks that seem too hard to do in one go, like writing a report or concentrating on bills, do them bit by bit, taking them on for a set period of time, say ten minutes, then have a break and do some more.

☺ Some things that help to reduce a craving for a cigarette are sweet or acid foods and beverages, and brief exercise (not exhaustive exercises). Therefore you can reduce cravings with citric fruits or juices. Rubbing a cut lemon over your tongue helps a craving.

☺ Don't fight a sweet tooth—there is a reason that you may have this. Glucose tablets (bought in any chemist) can help reduce the urge for sweet things, and artificial sweeteners are just as good. Chocolate has endorphins (the brain-calming chemical) in it, so it also helps. Don't panic that you will become a lolly eater instead of a cigarette smoker—this is a very short-term effect of quitting.

🚭 Try some *short* exercises, e.g. jog on the spot, push ups, run up and down the staircase each time you think 'I wouldn't mind a cigarette'. These are simple little exercises that you can do even at work. The important thing here is to get your heart rate up and some adrenalin released into your bloodstream. You'll feel as is if you've just had a cigarette.

🚭 Go a day at a time. 'Just for today I'll go without a cigarette.' Try not to project yourself too far ahead.

Category B
The smokers in this group may have known for a while that their need to smoke was somewhat different to other people who smoke. They may have attempted to quit in the past, achieved a day or two, perhaps longer and then succumbed to either the craving or some situation that triggered them off. All the tips for Category A apply to Category B smokers, but some form of nicotine replacement therapy would be needed as well. Currently, as mentioned before, there are two forms available, the Nicotine gum and the nicotine transdermal patch. Both of these are set courses that have to be followed. They should be taken seriously and followed through. It is like taking any course of medication for any other illness. Some of these replacement therapies are on prescription and you will need to see your doctor. Nicotine replacement therapies are currently contra-indicated in pregnancy. If you are pregnant see 'Pregnancy' at the end of this chapter. Reporting in to your doctor, especially

when you have quit smoking, can be an enormously encouraging step. Your doctor should be thrilled that you have made a serious decision to quit.

There are currently two forms of nicotine replacement therapy available. There is the Nicorette gum (Kabi Pharmacia) and the nicotine transdermal patches of which there are a variety: Nicotinel, Ciba-Geigy, Nicabate from Marion-Merrill-Dow and the Nicorette Patch by Kabi Pharmacia.

The principle behind all these therapies is the same. They all deliver a dose of nicotine that is *low* and *slow*. The graph demonstrates how the amount of nicotine derived from smoking compares with the amount derived from the gum and the patches.

What is outstandingly obvious is that with smoking there are the ups and downs of nicotine in the blood that are very distinct but with the others the line is straighter. The delivery of nicotine in these other forms does not hold within them the positive reinforcement that inhaling from a cigarette gives (see chapter 1). Contrary to what may people believe, they also do not deliver very much nicotine. However, they do give just enough to keep the cravings at bay.

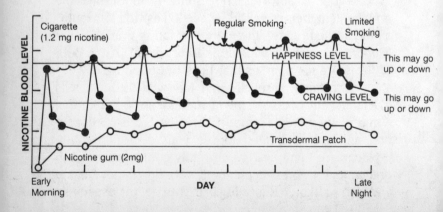

The idea then is that your nicotine cravings are taken care of while you take care of the psychological or behavioural aspects of smoking. Do you then become permanently hooked on the gum or the patch? The evidence is very strong that you won't if you use it correctly. Proper instructions on how to use the gum and patches have been given already.

Nicorette: Many smokers reading this may have attempted to use Nicorette in the past and decided that they didn't like it. In most cases the use was incorrect and if the instructions are correctly followed this therapy can be the mainstay of quitting. Read the instructions for use very carefully.

The nicotine tablet called Nicorette is a course that should cover at least six weeks, ideally twelve weeks. It is often hard to judge how long to go on using it as each individual varies, however the smoker using Nicorette should know to use it liberally. At first the need will be greater. Most smokers in Category B will need *at least* ten pieces of gum per day, some up to twenty, but as time goes by the need will diminish and so the usage will go down.

Nicorette helps those smokers who feel that they have a physical need to do something with their hands. The actual ritual of smoking can be transferred to the ritual of opening a packet of Nicorette tablets. There are many smokers who have tried using the 2 mg Nicorette and for a variety of reasons stopped taking it. They have complained it tasted bad, gave them hiccups or it stuck to their dentures. The major problems faced with Nicorette can be solved if it is used as follows:

⊛ Always start Nicorette first thing in the morning before getting out of bed. Sometimes you may need to use two gums to get started.

⊗ Don't chew it like chewing gum! The nicotine that you swallow with saliva is lost. The nicotine in the gum is absorbed through the lining of your mouth. Leave the gum in your mouth to work and bite it every now and then.

⊗ Use the gum as often as you think of having a cigarette— there's no limit to how many you can use or how often you use them.

⊗ Never drink fluids while the gum is in your mouth, or you wash the nicotine away. Use Nicorettes *before* your cup of coffee or tea, fruit juice etc.

⊗ Never wait till you are craving. The gum works slowly and will leave you dissatisfied if you wait too long.

⊗ Don't limit the quantity you use. After a few weeks you will automatically cut down without trying to. Let your need for nicotine dictate how much and how often you use Nicorettes in the first few weeks.

⊗ Always carry the gum with you, even months after you don't need it any more.

Take note: one 2 mg gum is roughly half to a third of a cigarette's worth of nicotine; and one 4 mg gum is the rough equivalent of one cigarette.

Most of the problems confronted with using Nicorette have to do with misuse of the gum. Here are some remedies to some of the typical problems:

Sticks to the denture: mix with Freedent non-stick chewing gum.
Hiccups: chewing too rapidly.
Acid stomach: chewing too rapidly.
Bad taste: mix with any other gum to improve flavour.
Gum's too soft: sticky from heat. Keep gums cool. Don't

carry them in your pocket, especially on hot days.

Mouth ulcers: not due to chewing Nicorette, but due to nicotine deprivation. Use more gum, not less.

If these instructions are followed then the smoker who is using Nicorette should feel as if they are smoking, only they're not. You shouldn't have any of those symptoms of withdrawal listed in chapter 1.

Transdermal nicotine patches: If you feel that the patch is easier for you because you hate the idea of putting things into your mouth regularly or you're embarrassed to be seen with gum, then this is ideal. The patches are changed every day but the length of time you use the patch depends on the brand of patch you buy. Most manufacturers recommend that they are worn for a minimum six to nine weeks. Because there are a variety of these patches and because they are on prescription only at the moment, your doctor is best equipped to discuss with you which one should be used. However, there have been some common problems. The patches that are worn overnight are made so that a relatively high blood level is available to the smoker when they wake up. This is to avoid the early morning cigarette and thus the cycle of ups and downs that would then ensue. Because there is a slow release of nicotine through the patch at night some smokers have found their sleep can be disturbed. They may, in particular, have vivid dreams.

Once you commence on this sort of therapy it is not enough to be reliant on this and nothing else—though you must cover the course completely.

Category C
If you have found yourself in this category do not despair! You would imagine, and it may have been so in the

past, that things will be too tough and you may as well forget about being able to quit. This is not the case at all! We know that your need to smoke is very much bound up with the amount of nicotine in your bloodstream, which is probably higher than the other categories. Replacing the nicotine with another form of it is ideal in your case, but you will need a strong dose. Follow the instructions for Category B, but there will be a need to have some form or nicotine replacement therapy as well. The nicotine patches developed so far may not deliver sufficient nicotine to satisfy you and it is not recommended that you use them in the first instance. You may have had past experience using Nicorette but this time you will require the 4 mg concentration for which you will need a doctor's prescription.

Before you begin, however, if you are smoking more than 30 cigarettes a day it is a good idea to keep a record of your smoking every day for three days. (See the chart.) You should start in the morning and note what time you light a cigarette and what you are doing for every single cigarette you have for three days. Don't write down you have, say, five together. Each cigarette has to be accounted for separately. The reason for doing this is not always self-evident. Look at the time intervals between your cigarettes. You may notice they are very distinct, like clockwork. This is also an indication of how often you're going to have to have a new piece of Nicorette. Just keeping a record of your smoking if you smoke more than 30 a day will reduce the amount you smoke spontaneously. After the third day, start the 4 mg Nicorette on the morning of the fourth day. It is advised that you use just as much as you need in the beginning. There may be a need to use it hourly, which is fine. Do not be concerned that this is a permanent need. It will be reduced in time.

Cigarette Tally Sheet

Day			Day	
No.	Time	Occasion	Time	Occasion
1				
2				
3				
4				
5				
6				
7				
8				
9				
10				
11				
12				
13				
14				
15				
16				
17				
18				
19				
20				
21				
22				
23				
24				
25				
26				
27				
28				
29				
30				
31				
32				
33				
34				
35				
36				
37				
38				
39				
40				

Special cases

Pregnancy

One in three pregnant women smoke. The numbers will increase as there are so many young girls in our society that smoke. These young women often promise themselves that they will not smoke when they get pregnant but unfortunately by this time they are well and truly hooked. You would expect that just the notion that you are pregnant is enough to help you quit. It isn't quite like that.

Ethically the objective here in smoking cessation is to help the person who wishes to quit to do so for themselves, but the perspective is different if there is a foetus involved. Lumbering a woman with the guilt of smoking is not very productive as the anxiety caused by this may even cause her to smoke more. However, the foetus is the most intensively involved passive smoker. Since it receives the same blood as the mother, nicotine and the destructive carbon monoxide also pass into the bloodstream of the baby. The effect on the foetus are huge. From conception to delivery women who smoke have:

- A reduced fertility.

- Increased risk of bleeding in pregnancy.

- Highest risk of spontaneous abortion.

- Low birth weight babies.

- Babies with an increased risk of birth defects.

Quitting in the first three months of pregnancy protects the foetus from all of the above. Reducing cigarette intake has little benefit.

The ironical situation exists today that a woman who

is pregnant and dependent on nicotine is unable to have nicotine replacement therapy prescribed to her, as nicotine is classed as a poison and contraindicated in pregnancy. Of course that same woman can buy nicotine at her local grocer. Those women who have tested themselves in chapter 2 may have found ways to help themselves quit. If however the dependency is severe, withdrawals may be very strong and the ability to remain abstinent becomes very difficult. The information in chapter 4 may be helpful. Also use the 14-day reduction plan to quit, at the end of this chapter.

Adolescents
There is no reason why young people who smoke should not be as addicted as adults who smoke. The addiction does not take years to acquire, just as tolerance to the side effects of smoking does not take years. It seems that adolescents can have as difficult a time in quitting as adults. The difference is that many kids don't try to quit so they don't know they have a problem with it. It is only when they make an attempt to not smoke for a while they notice that their smoking is not a random, controllable event. They are often under the impression that they can take it or leave it and will often lie to their elders about this. Rather than badger a young smoker about their future illness, which is as remote to them as the moon, a good ploy with an adolescent is to suggest to them that perhaps they are hooked. Most will vigorously deny this. Then suggest that if they are not hooked they should be able to go at least a week without a cigarette. Some will notice that they find this quite difficult. The whole concept of being addicted to cigarettes usually never occurs to them. The other concern, particularly of adults and teachers is what to do about a child who smokes and is caught openly.

Most adults are distressed by this even if they themselves are smokers. Nothing is more ludicrous than an adult coming up to a schoolkid and telling them 'Don't smoke, you'll regret it like I do.'

Studies have shown that if these children are given an open policy on their smoking they will use it liberally and are more likely to become full on adult smokers. If, however, their smoking is very restricted (this means no smoking in the house, no special rooms set aside to smoke etc.) these adolescents are less likely to become adult smokers. This may seem Draconian, but seems to work in many cases. It's rather the 'give them a hand, they'll take your whole arm.'

Of course it is implicit in the above discussion that kids have access to tobacco, which they undoubtably have, though it is against the law not only to sell cigarettes to any person under the age of 18 but to even 'provide' them with one.

Coronary artery disease and other medical complications
Again the irony is that these smokers are expected to have quit smoking because they have had a life-threatening illness. It is assumed by many that this is sufficient motivation to quit. This is not necessarily so. We have studied patients about to undergo open heart surgery and found 10 per cent were smoking the day before the operation. These 10 per cent were lying about their smoking status to all the medical staff. But because we have a better understanding of the nature of addictions we know why people would do this. An addiction overrides all rational thought. Especially in a stressful situation, a smoker is much more likely to need a cigarette than not. If a smoker is in the category of severe dependency and their doctor cannot recommend

nicotine replacement therapy then the method mentioned below may help.

At the end of this chapter a set program that was devised many years ago to help smokers who are either pregnant or have had medical complications whereby they are unable to use nicotine replacement therapies. The program goes over fourteen days. It is a tapering procedure where you are rationed so many cigarettes per day, not unlike a diet.

Psychiatric illnesses
It is anecdotal that a very large proportion of the psychiatrically ill smoke. Smoking occurs in many with severe depression, the anxiety disorders and in mostly all schizophrenics. Why such a high proportion? There is evidence that these smokers may be smoking to relieve their symptoms. Certainly their symptoms get considerably worse when they attempt to quit, which can often be the cause of their relapsing. Smokers like this are often given cigarettes to 'help them along' by well-meaning family or hospital staff. Unfortunately the physical effects from smoking do not spare the psychiatrically ill. Some are keen to quit and make attempts to do so with great enthusiasm. This enthusiasm is often short lived when, for example, manic depressives are then suddenly thrown into the chasm of black depression, which is a common withdrawal symptom. They immediately resort to smoking. Little work has been done to date to assess the level of dependency in the majority of these patients, however it is conceivable that most would be highly dependent. If this is so, it is interesting to look at the combination of nicotine addiction, which we know is neurochemical, and these illnesses, which are also often neurochemical in origin. The treatment in these cases would be the same for

any person highly dependent: nicotine replacement in almost all cases, depending on the patient's own co-operation, ability and stability. These patients would need to be monitored by their physicians throughout to control any exacerbation of their disease.

Abstinent alcoholics and other drug users
These are a group of people that are invariably heavily addicted smokers. Many wish to be totally drug free and have a very good perception of their addiction to nico-tine, having had the experience of other drugs. Our experiences with this type of smoker is that they do very well in quitting as they understand the notions of withdrawals and coping with temptations. Some 'dry' alcoholics who have attended Alcoholics Anonymous have put their smoking 'on the program' and have had success doing this.

Fourteen day reduction to quit plan
As mentioned before, cutting down is not the objective as most smokers find this difficult to maintain and usually compensate by inhaling deeper and smoking more of the actual cigarette. Cutting out *altogether* is the aim. The method described below is used in cases were smokers find it either uncomfortable to quit cold turkey or cannot commence nicotine replacement therapy as it is contra-indicated in their medical condition.

You begin this method by keeping a record of your actual normal smoking for three days. Use the record chart. This gives you an accurate account of the number you smoke and from the average you can then calculate how many cigarettes you reduce by every day. The actual reduction begins on the fourth day. For each day you have a ration of cigarettes from which you must not deviate. It is best to take out the ration for the day and put it in a container like a plastic bag. Follow the guide day by day through the programme. When you have achieved the last day then go on to chapter 4 for continued help into the first few days of quitting.

Your ration
For example, if you smoke an average of 16–25 a day you are to take 18 cigarettes with you. Those 18 cigarettes, or 45 if you smoke 46–55 a day, are going to be your ration tomorrow through the day, but remember from your tally sheets, keep cigarettes for the end of the day too.

Ration Reckoner for Tapering

Daily Average	0–15	16–25	26–35	36–45	46–55	56–65	66–75
Day 5	9	18	27	36	45	54	63
Day 6	8	16	24	32	40	48	56
Day 7	7	14	21	28	35	42	49
Day 8	6	12	18	24	30	36	42
Day 9	5	10	15	20	25	30	35
Day 10	4	8	12	16	20	24	28
Day 11	3	6	9	12	15	18	21
Day 12	2	4	6	8	10	12	14
Day 13	1	2	3	4	5	6	7

Day 14—Attempt 24 hrs without a cigarette

☒ 4 ☒

Troubleshooting in the first few days

New ex-smokers will have the same common problems no matter which method they have chosen to quit.

After a few days have gone by without a cigarette many new quitters have no idea what to expect next. 'Will I be like this the rest of my life?' Others who have had a relatively easy time of it are waiting for the crunch to come. Whatever the reactions are, your obsessions with smoking will slow down eventually.

You may now be priding yourself on the achievement of having gone a few days without a cigarette. *There is everything to be proud of.* No one gives credit to how difficult quitting is for some smokers. Nicotine is one of the most addictive substances known to humankind but most people have no sympathy.

Surviving the first few days
Like all other drugs of addiction there is a great attraction to have just one because you've achieved some time without one. The last thing you should do is reward yourself with the substance that you are trying not to

use. Reward yourself with anything else you can think of except a cigarette.

Ninety-five per cent of smokers who have a lapse (this means one cigarette) while they are trying to quit relapse. It is vital to understand that a single cigarette is a major concern and should not be dismissed as a minor event. *Quitting counts from the last cigarette you had.*

As mentioned before, the unfortunate truth about stopping smoking is that nobody has much sympathy for you. You're expected to tough this out on your own. Heroin addicts going cold turkey are allowed to sweat it out and there is even a romanticised view of them having their withdrawals while some concerned loved one mops their brow. No one would ever expect them to go to work, cook meals, or carry on with life normally. However, society expects that coming off nicotine is easy and you are to carry on as normal.

What causes relapse in the first two weeks?
The graph shows the likelihood of relapse in the first two weeks of quitting among smokers who receive no help. Your objective now is to achieve two weeks without smoking and not become one of the statistics in the graph.

What were the main reasons these smokers relapsed in the first two weeks?

1. They lacked commitment and confidence.
2. They drank alcohol.
3. They were living with a smoker or someone very close to them was a smoker.

What does *not* count in the relapse in the first two weeks was how old you are, how many cigarettes a day you smoked or whether you are male or female. This means

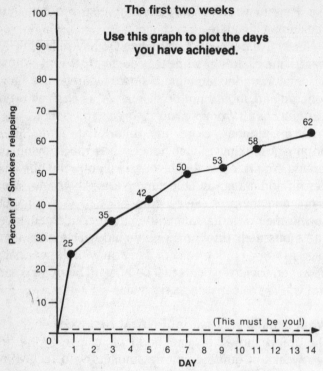

This graph show that 62% of smokers who do not have any help relapse in the first two weeks. Your goal is to get past the first two weeks.

the three main causes of relapse in the first two weeks are elements that you are well capable of arranging for yourself.

1. You will have made a strong and solid decision to do something about your smoking or you would not be this far into reading this book. Your confidence in your ability naturally waxes and wanes but with a better understanding of your dependency you will now be able to tackle this in a very different way than

you have ever done before. Commitment to quit can be lost in an instant of emotional upset. If conditions around you are more distressing than usual, it is worthwhile remembering that anxiety and tension is a symptom of withdrawal and that you may be over-reacting to these situations. It may seem that everybody is getting on your nerves intentionally. This over-reaction does go away but you must let it happen. If you find that you are overly distressed there are many excellent relaxation tapes that are available. The technique usually used is progressive muscle tension and relaxation. A tape can be played just about anywhere, in the car, at home or at work in your break. It is an excellent diversion from the circumstances around you.

2. You should be able to avoid all alcohol for two weeks. If you cannot, then you may have to seriously consider whether you have a problem with alcohol. Some people may think that not drinking for this length of time is outrageous, however if your commitment to quit smoking is real, then the advice is DO NOT DRINK. This is after all not a permanent state; you will be able to go back to drinking moderately after this time.

3. Living with a smoker is a problem that at first seems insurmountable because if your husband or wife smokes you can hardly separate from each other because of it. If a very close friend who you are often with smokes, it can also be the cause of relapse. You are not expected to give up your friend. There is no need to ram quitting down their throats either because that only antagonises the situation. However, a reasonable rearrangement can be found for these situations. *Inhaling* the cigarette smoke is as important a component of your need to smoke when someone else is smoking. *Seeing* them do it is less important.

The best solution is if that person wants to smoke, which is after all their perogative, then either you leave the room or they should while it's happening. There is no need to antagonise another smoker, but do make a physical move.

Small enclosed spaces like cars do present a difficulty. If it's your car then you call the shots—'No smoking in my car'—but if it's not yours then you may have to make it clear that you're very allergic to cigarette smoke right now (not altogether untrue!).

Fitting in
What to do with your hands
A smoker puts their hand to their mouth about 200 times a day. There will now have to be 200 other ways you

> YOUR LUNGS DO NOT SLOWLY FILL UP WITH TAR IN WHICH YOU WILL EVENTUALLY DROWN.

will have to deal with your hands. This is not as serious a problem as it may seem. Many smokers, when they first think about quitting, think that the handling of a cigarette, lighting it up, seeing the smoke rise is a very important component of smoking. Fortunately it is not that important as you will notice once you are not smoking. If it is something that is a problem then an activity that involves both hands and head is ideal. You don't have to be any good at it. For example, if you have never knitted, both males or females can practise knitting as it takes up not only your hands but your head as well.

Other people smoking
When you're trying not to smoke you have a tendency to become obsessed with other people smoking. You

notice every smoker. It seems that when you were smoking no one else did it; now that you're not, everyone else is. They cannot both be true. Be aware that this is a passing distortion of what is really going on. You will soon lose your interest in them.

Offers to smoke

Some new non-smokers have to get used to the idea of not doing it any more. If you are famous in your group for smoking and now you don't want to do it any more the best way to fend off other people offering you a cigarette is to not draw attention to yourself. If you are offered a cigarette don't say 'I'm trying to quit', say 'Not right now' or even 'I just had one, thanks'. This takes the heat off you. This way there is no dialogue entered into as to what, where, how and why you're not smoking.

Withdrawals

What can be done about the symptoms of withdrawal? All of them are due to nicotine deprivation. How long can they be expected to last? If you are using a nicotine replacement therapy, these reactions should be occurring minimally. If they are happening then increase the amount or dose you are using as well as follow some of the advice given on how to deal with them.

Many studies carried out on the time course of withdrawals have come to show that they can range from four days to about five weeks. This does not mean that you will have to deal with them each day, all day over this time period. These symptoms dissipate over the five-week period until they are no longer felt.

Cravings
Anxiety
Irritability

Lack of concentration
Nervousness, tension
Hypersomnia/Insomnia
Hyperactivity
Aggression
Headaches
Cramps
Light-headedness
Constipation
Increase of appetite, especially for sweet foods

Cravings
No one knows exactly what a craving is. It's not something that can easily be measured like blood pressure or temperature. It is an overwhelming need to . . . or a strong desire to have . . . X. What we do know is that the intensity and duration of the cravings diminish with time. Some people feel that a craving seems to last all day long, while others have a 'bolt of lightning' type of craving that is gone very quickly. It is often a good idea to time your cravings by your watch. Exactly how long do they last? Count them too. How many a day do you really have? You can even compare the days. Being aware that there will be less and less of them and that they don't last very long will help. The most important thing is to realise that they will eventually abate.

If as part of a craving you get a 'taste' for a cigarette in your mouth, a slice of lemon rubbed across the tongue gets rid of this almost immediately.

Anxiety, tension, light-headedness, headaches and a sweet tooth
As mentioned in chapter 1, the anxiety and irritability that you may be experiencing is a symptom of withdrawals and is not a 'new' you. Your personality is not

likely to change permanently. These are transient effects from nicotine deprivation and you must recognise them for what they are. They are so transient that they usually last a maximum of four days.

It seems one of the main causes of anxiety and tension is due to a drop in blood sugar level that can occur when you stop smoking. This is also the reason some people get light-headed and have a sweet tooth when they have just stopped. An increase in glucose intake can have a positive effect on all these symptoms. Glucose in either tablet or powder form is ideal but needs to be taken several times a day for the first few days. We have glucose jelly beans on hand in our clinic at all

---

CIGARS ARE NOT BETTER FOR YOU. SOME CIGARS CONTAIN TOXIC LEVELS OF NICOTINE. AN UNLIT CIGAR CAN ALSO GIVE HIGH NICOTINE WHILE IT'S CHEWED ON.

---

times for this reason. They can quite distinctly alter someone's bad mood when they come into the clinic!

Another very recent and most unusual finding in smokers is the effect coffee has on withdrawals. We know that caffeine levels are reduced when you smoke. When you quit, if you are used to several cups of coffee a day or more you may become caffeine intoxicated. The symptoms of caffeine intoxication are nervousness, anxiety and irritability, very similar to nicotine withdrawals. Take care of your coffee intake by reducing it by half, though you may find that your interest in coffee has decreased spontaneously.

Aggression
The link between aggression and tension and anxiety is very strong. This can be very real and frightening for

some people who are otherwise quiet, passive types. The tips described above, reducing caffeine intake, and increasing glucose intake, may help.

Constipation

This is often the unmentionable symptom. No one wants to admit to having a cigarette on the toilet in the morning to get their bowels moving, but many people have done this. It is believed that nicotine affects bowel activity. With nicotine withdrawn there is a slowing down of activity. If this is occurring then it's better to increase the fibre in your diet for a while.

Hypersomnia or insomnia

These are both classic symptoms of withdrawals from many drugs. Being very sleepy is due to the lack of nicotine, which is a pep-up type of drug. The need to sleep excessively then causes insomnia afterwards. This usually lasts only a few days and then tends to straighten out into your normal routine. It is strongly advised not to take sleeping tablets at this time.

Hyperactivity

Some smokers when they have quit react by becoming hyped up. They rush around furiously doing things. This may be a type of conscious way of distraction, but is probably more likely to be a chemical reaction. This may occur due to the caffeine toxicity effect, but the need to keep busy, passing time, is inherent in the problem of quitting.

If any of these symptoms are particularly strong and you feel that the temptations to smoke to overcome them are very strong, then you should consider going up one category or reassessing yourself and your level of dependency. Particularly those in Category A. They may find that they need to go to Category B. The categories are a guideline only but sometimes withdrawals are stronger than expected for the category you are in.

The method you have chosen to help you stop smoking should reduce the withdrawals to a minimum. Ideally you should have none at all. *Change tactics straight away* if you feel that what you are doing is ineffective and you have followed all the instructions (including the one about no alcohol).

Time

Accruing time behind you without smoking is one of the most important aspects in the first days. This may seem self-evident but the longer you go without smoking the longer you'll go without smoking.

Time itself seems longer when you are trying not to smoke. One minute passing is like an hour to some. The activity of smoking does take up an inordinate amount of time. Especially today, where you may be in an office or workplace where you may not smoke, you have to leave the premises to do it, all of which takes time. But sitting down and relaxing with a cigarette also takes in time. Now you are left with this extra time. Keep active and busy distracting yourself. Sitting twiddling your thumbs saying to yourself 'It'll go away' is about the worst thing you can do.

☺ 5 ☺

Troubleshooting: the bigger picture

Many days may now have gone by without smoking. There should be a feeling of great achievement. To have been able to overcome a drug like nicotine with its strong potency is a major accomplishment.

No matter what category you are in on the dependency scale the problems of long-term quitting become the same for all new ex-smokers.

Here is where the plot thickens. More often than not the feelings of withdrawal are less frequent, cravings are getting less if not gone altogether. Some new quitters are so laid back that it's a surprise to them. They may suddenly experience a calmness that they have rarely had before. This is because they are out of the cycle of withdrawals they were in when they were smokers.

What may occur is some quitters however is the insidious part of smoking cessation called JUSTIFYING HAVING A CIGARETTE. It is as if the brain, having given up trying to get at you with physical withdrawals, tries a new tactic and tries to get at you through your thoughts. You may begin rationalising some of these things:

1. I have this whole thing under control, I can do this any time I like.
2. I'll have just one whenever I like.
3. I can't see any immediate physical improvement . . . what's the point of quitting?
4. Smoking after all never affected my health, now I know I can do it, I'll quit like this if I get sick, pregnant etc.
5. I'm sick of this . . . I don't need the gum or the patch any more.

These thoughts are called 'Stinking Thinking' in Alcoholics Anonymous, and the same should apply to nicotine addicts. On the one shoulder sits the angel that is encouraging you to stay stopped, and on the other shoulder sits the devil saying 'Go on, one won't hurt.'

The ideas listed above seem rational enough but:

1. If you could have had this under control you would have years ago.
2. Having just one is the major cause of relapse. There are two reasons for this. One is that the nicotine enters your bloodstream, going rapidly to your brain cells, once again turning them on. The second reason is that when you have had one cigarette you often get so demoralised when you realise what you've done that you immediately give up giving up.
3 and 4. There is an expectation that you will be brilliantly well almost immediately after quitting. You cannot expect an instant effect. Some people do have a very quick reaction but others feel a slow and gradual improvement. Whatever the reaction is, it's a good one. The physical effects of quittting are so profound that chaper 6 has been devoted entirely to it. It is worthwhile turning to it now if you feel your motivations are slipping.

5. A common reaction to using the nicotine replacement therapies is to decide that you don't need them any more now that a certain amount of time has passed. There may be a fear that you will become dependent on the therapy or again that you simply don't need it any more. These are fatal errors to make. The therapy should be carried out to its full course and not any shorter than that.

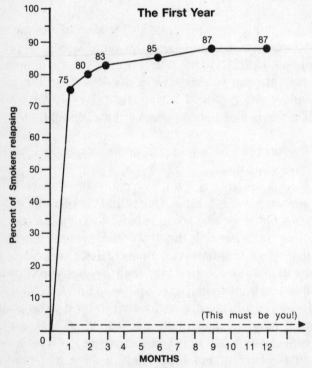

This graph shows that most smokers relapse within the first three months. Therefore your goal is three months.

The graph shows a fuller picture in time than the one shown in chapter 4. As you can see this gives a view to the future. The future has a deadline: it is three months. Why are three months of abstinence so important? Once three months has been achieved the likelihood of relapse is very low. No one seems to know why this is an important time frame for those wanting to stay stopped. It is possible that it takes the nicotine receptor sites in the brain this long to properly adapt. However, what is striking about this time frame is that it follows very closely the time frame of grieving. Like the loss of a loved one.

Some longer-term syptoms of withdrawal
Forgetfulness
Grief
Depression
Curiosity about using again
Cough
Mouth ulcers

As mentioned before, these symptoms don't always occur, and if the method used to help you stop smoking have been properly adhered to they should be minimal.

Forgetfulness
This of course doesn't mean that you forget who you are; it is mostly a vagueness that can be quite irritating, like forgetting where you've put things etc. This may take some time to staighten out but is quite normal and very much due to nicotine deprivation.

Grief
It is not an exaggeration that many smokers complain that the loss of their smoking is likened to the loss of a loved one. Though no scientific analysis has been carried out on this sensation to date, it is interesting

to note that these sensations diminish in time parallel with the grief process experienced by those in mourning.

Grief over the loss of cigarettes is a common complaint and should not be dismissed as insignificant. It can be so real in fact that another common manifestation of grief can occur, and that is dreaming about smoking. Some people, after weeks of not smoking, suddenly wake up in a panic sweat absolutely sure that they smoked. They are very relieved when they realised that they were dreaming.

Depression
Only very recently have investigators looked at the notion that some smokers may be smoking to suppress symptoms of depression. It may well be that the smoking itself is the cause of the depression. There are cases of patients with a past history of clinical depression relieving their symptoms by smoking. This is unusual in non-depressed smokers but medical advice needs to be sought if the depression is considered too great. Depression should not be confused with general unhappiness about not smoking.

Curiosity about using again
This reaction is common to all drug users who have stopped for a while. It usually goes, 'I wonder what it's like to have one again?' This is linked to missing the cigarettes and grieving over their loss. Unfortunately newly quit smokers have a problem in that the drug they were dependent on is so readily accessible. Unlike a loved one who has gone, cigarettes are retrievable, you can buy them back in your local grocer shop.

Cough and mouth ulcers
These are two physical effects that some may see as

particularly negative. How is it that you can develop a cough when you quit? You may never have had a smoker's cough in your life! The cough is a good healthy clearance mechanism and may take a few weeks to clear.

Mouth ulcers are an even stranger reaction to quitting. They occur in about one in three smokers who quit. They are a symptom of withdrawal and do not last very long. They are not due to infection, poor diet or using the gum, but are more likely due to the distress of quitting. In fact if those using the gum have developed ulcers they should *increase* the amount they are using and the ulcers will go away.

If all is well and you have few of the sensations listed above there are only two events that may undo a new quitter in the near future. One there is control over and the other there is none.
1. You drink in excess and you have no control over what you are doing; or
2. A major crisis occurs and you instinctively reach for a cigarette.

Alcohol
We are aware alcohol and nicotine have a profound effect on each other. Now that some time has passed and you would like to drink again you must be wary of the effect of alcohol now that you don't smoke. It will be much more potent than before. You will get a stronger effect from drinking than you had when you were smoking. In fact you will soon notice that the 'morning after the night before' is mainly due to smoking and drinking together, and not so much a cause of drinking.

If you would like to drink again then the best advice is to drink your first glass of alcohol (only one) somewhere where there is definitely no threat of smoking around you. DO NOT GO TO THE CLUB OR PUB for your first drink after you've stopped smoking. Practise drinking at home first, and always in moderation.

A major crisis

Again, a major crisis to some is a minor one to others. However, there are events over which you have no control. If, for example, you receive a huge telephone bill, this may be an unexpected major crisis that makes you very nervous. You may instinctively want a cigarette.

Whatever the crisis it, it will not change if you smoke. The phone bill will not drop by one dollar if you do. It is impossible to anticipate or practice your reactions in a major crisis but it can come in handy if you think about how you would react if something serious did happen. Again you must be absolutely aware that even in these circumstances a lapse into smoking means a relapse.

How then do you get over a major crisis and not smoke? How do other people who've never smoked react to a major setback? The natural physical reaction to an adverse event for anybody is to be nervous and startled, to get a rise in blood pressure and increased heart rate and perhaps to hyperventilate. Recovery from this is relatively quick in that after about three to five minutes these reactions begin to fade. A smoker naturally reaches for a cigarette immediately so that the recovery period is equated with the use of the cigarette. The recovery period always occurs even if you don't smoke, but smokers don't know this. For example, if you don't smoke and you get angry with someone or something then the reaction would be to 'explode', then perhaps walk away or sit somewhere to cool off. A new quitter has to learn to do this. This again is a time element. Only the passing of days and then weeks will teach you to accommodate to these events like any non-smoker.

Learning how to behave

The instinct to smoke

How long does it take to learn how to behave without smoking? We have conducted some research on this subject and the results have been interesting. The instinctive reactions that smokers have to light up a cigarette in tempting situations goes away relatively quickly. In fact the more often these tempting situations occur and you don't smoke, the quicker your instinctive reaction to smoke goes away. An insight into this phenomenon is best understood using the example of Pavlovian conditioning.

Pavlovian conditioning: Some instinctive reactions are due to what is called in psychology Pavlovian conditioning. Ivan Pavlov was a Nobel prizewinning gastroenterologist in the 1920s. The conditioning response that he first described was an incidental discovery that he made while working on saliva. He had been studying saliva and gastric juices, wondering why they were produced, what they were chemically made of and how much was made. To better study saliva, he arranged some experiments where he had bags attached to the jaws of dogs, as dogs are famous for salivating a lot. He was measuring the amount and content of the saliva he collected and had several dogs rigged up like this. It was a busy laboratory and people were going in and out all the time. Pavlov noticed that when one person, an attendant, came into the laboratory all the dogs would be up on their hind legs yapping and producing copious amounts of saliva. This didn't happen if anybody else came in. What did this attendant do that nobody else did? This attendant fed the dogs. Pavlov immediately realised that the dogs had associated the attendant with food and when he came in to the laboratory they got

---

'MILD' LOW TAR, LOW NICOTINE CIGARETTES ARE NOT BETTER FOR YOU. THE LEVELS ARE SO LOW THAT SMOKERS WILL DRAG HARDER AND SO INHALE MORE CARBON MONOXIDE THAN EVER. THEY ARE THUS MUCH WORSE FOR YOU.

---

ready to eat and digest when they saw him, even if he had no food with him. They had an anticipatory reaction.

On the basis of this observation Pavlov set up a series of experiments. Firstly he had a bell (the cue) placed in front of the dog. When the bell rang the dog would be fed. Very quickly the dog learned that a bell ringing meant food was coming and would begin to salivate whenever the bell rang. Even if the bell rang and no food was placed in front of the dog, the dog would still salivate *in anticipation* of being fed. This learned reaction is called conditioning, the physical reaction in antici-pation of a reward, even though it may not occur.

If the dog is not fed every time the bell rings, it goes on salivating each time anyway . . . for a while. Then the dog starts to catch on, 'What's the point of salivating, getting ready to digest, if I don't get any food?' So the dog eventually stops salivating every time the bell rings and just ignores it. This is called extinguishing the response.

Next Pavlov thought, 'What would happen if I randomly fed the dog, sometimes yes, sometimes no, every now and again?' Of course the dog had no idea what would happen next; it may or may not get fed on the next bell ringing, or maybe only on the twentieth bell ring. The dog will go on salivating every time, just in case it gets the reward of food and needs to digest it. This randomised rewarding perpetuates the reaction.

The lessons to be learnt from Pavlov's dogs are very important in addictions and the positive reinforcements that they elicit. Smoking can easily be seen in the same light. Humans are considered more sophisticated than dogs, and their cues are therefore more sophisticated. In smoking, the bell ringing (the cue) can be the telephone, driving the car, an argument, a meal, coffee, sex etc. All of these activities are equated with smoking. If we look closely at Pavlov's work we know that if you ring the bell (the cue) repeatedly and don't feed the dog, the dogs stops reacting. This also occurs in smoking. If you allow the cue, say having a cup of coffee, to occur and don't smoke, the more often you have that coffee the quicker you will not react to it with a need to smoke. Therefore avoidance of these cues is not recommended. *Do not avoid doing what you always did.* You may already notice that you can in fact answer the phone now very easily without smoking. This is because answering the phone may be something you do very frequently, and so the instinctive reaction to smoke wears off very quickly. The more frequent the event the quicker it wears off. This doesn't mean that you should pick a fight several times a day so that you can rid yourself of the instinct to smoke after a fight, but it does mean that these cues that trigger an urge to smoke wear away with time as long as you do not reward the urge.

It is important to note that none of this applies to alcohol. I have explained before that alcohol has a chemical effect on the brain cells altogether unrelated to this. Therefore frequent drinking for this cue is not the answer!

Not all new quitters, however, are triggered off by cues. Some just get an urge to smoke out of the blue for what seems to be no good reason. It is often a 'miss it' sensation that then goes away. Again, all these sensations are taken care of with time. There should be less and less of the need to smoke, or of missing it, as time passes.

The great weight gain debate

If ever there was a put off to quitting smoking it is the fear of weight gain. Both women and men believe that they will put on weight if they stop smoking, but because of complex pressures placed on them in our society, women come close to paranoia about it. Most people have no real experience of gaining weight when they quit, but will continue to complain that it may be so or that they know someone who did, which justifies their attitude. The excuse that weight gain will be medically detrimental is also well used but misinformed. Many young women are fostered with this opinion and begin smoking to remain slim, with no evidence whatsoever that they would not have remained slim without it.

The general scientific concensus is that the weight gain associated with smoking cessation is minimal and poses no health consequences. It is estimated that about half of all quitters will gain some weight and the average gain is about 2.3 kilograms.

What is interesting is that this weight gain that does occur doesn't seem to generate relapse. Though it is a big fear and causes a wide amount of discussion before and after quitting it is a weak cause of relapsing to smoking. What is the cause of some of this weight gain? It has been hypothesised that it is due to the increase in food intake and reduction in metabolic rate. In those smokers where nicotine replacement therapy is used, weight gain does not seem to occur at all. Therefore nicotine per se seems to be implicated in the effect.

Should you diet while you're quitting? Or how long

afterwards should you start? It is not recommended that you diet vigorously when you're quitting smoking. Like any other endeavour, the focus of attention should be on not smoking and not on anything else. Dealing with too many NOs can be too stressful and ultimately counterproductive. Three months should pass before you consider a change in eating habits. By then any other effects from not smoking may also have taken place, like an increase in ability to exercise or simply doing things. Both these effects stimulate appetite but also help weight control, so it is best to wait and see what happens.

☺ **6** ☺

The physical effects of quitting

In the past thirty years there have been literally tens of thousands of medical articles written on the health consequences of smoking. No educated person can ignore or dispute the evidence. But what happens when a person quits smoking? What are the benefits to them then? Is the damage irreparable?

The major conclusions from the research are that smoking cessation immediately benefits all smokers no matter what their age or whether they have or do not have a smoking-related illness.

Risk of getting sick from smoking once you've stopped

There is a difference between getting sick from the actual inhalation of a chemical and the *risk* of getting sick and dying from it. Two out of four smokers die from their smoking. Not everyone does. Why do some and not others?

It is interesting to note that there are so many diseases we know that are caused by smoking like lung cancer, heart disease, emphysema, vascular disease, and ulcers, it is surprising that not everybody gets all of them. Most people do not even get some of them but a lot of people get one of them.

The basis for the selection of who is going to die and who is going to get sick and who is not going to get anything at all from smoking are luck and risk factors. We know, for example, that if you have a family history of heart attacks, if your blood cholesterol is high and if you smoke, altogether you run a very grave risk of having a fatal heart attack. If you take away the cholesterol and the family history, smoking is still the *major* risk factor for heart disease. The risk factors for emphysema are also high if there is a family history of lung disease, especially bronchitis and asthma. Though not everyone who has these diseases has any family history of them at all. In the end it's the luck of the draw, and how you chose your parents. You may not have ever got sick from smoking but what all this means is that giving up smoking has a hugely positive effect on your well-being. For example, if you quit smoking before the age of 50 you will reduce the risk of dying in the next fifteen years by half.

What if you are sick from smoking, if you already do have heart disease or emphysema or a stomach ulcer? Then basically the effects are the same. The heart improves and so do the lungs. The ulcers heal. Nothing deteriorates, that is, even the emphysema does not get worse if you stop smoking.

What happens to the chemicals once you quit smoking?

Over 4000 chemicals have been identified in tobacco smoke. The body is profoundly affected by this personal pollution but has a repair capacity that is astounding. This repair has been going on all the time someone smokes. In fact, if this was not so, cigarette smoking would have killed a new smoker very quickly. Even within the first few months, when you had just begun to smoke, mechanisms to clear away the chemicals had already begun to work.

The biggest myth that abounds about smoking is that chemicals from smoking are stored in the body. People are under the impression that it may take as many years as the person has smoked to get all the chemicals out. They think that if you have been smoking for twenty years then it will take twenty years for all the chemicals to be washed out of the body. There is absolutely no basis for this belief at all. The evidence to date show that by four months after quitting there are no remnants or by-products remaining in the body. This may seem fast but in biological terms it is very slow.

Not all the chemicals inhaled actually pass into the bloodstream. In fact 80 per cent of what is inhaled is exhaled immediately into the air. Film of smoke being inhaled looks like a snow storm in the lungs, with particles flying all over the place which then finally settle down on to the lining of the lungs. Some chemicals are in gas form and pass straight through the lung into the bloodstream. Nicotine for example goes through into the lung vaporised due to the heat of smoking. It then mixes into the blood and circulates. There are many thousands of chemicals in the tobacco smoke, but some seem to be more important than others and the indications are that they are responsible for the illnesses we know about today.

Carbon monoxide
The substance considered to be the most dangerous in smoking is the gas carbon monoxide (CO). This gas can occur naturally from any type of burning or

combustion. It is produced in fires, in car exhausts and from smoking. It is odourless and tasteless and gives no warning of its presence. The concentration from smoking is very very high, much higher than would be imagined, and this is because smoking goes on right at the mouth and straight undiluted into the lungs. Even car exhaust is diluted by the atmosphere in the open air, so that the excuse given by many smokers that the level of carbon monoxide they have from smoking is lower than from the traffic in the street is untrue.

Why is this gas so dangerous? The unfortunate situation is that this gas is readily taken up into the blood's red cells. Their job normally is to carry and distribute oxygen. The red cells circulate around the body picking

> THE CARBON MONOXIDE INHALED FROM CAR EXHAUST IN THE STREET IS NOWHERE NEAR AS HIGH AS THE CARBON MONOXIDE INHALED FROM A CIGARETTE.

up oxygen from the lungs and delivering it to the rest of the body. When carbon monoxide comes into the lungs from inhaling a cigarette, that gas gets preference over oxygen, where the red cells absorb the carbon monoxide 200 times more avidly than even oxygen. What then occurs is that this gas circulates around the bloodstream bound up in the red cells. The red cells then cannot do their normal carrying job. Every inhalation from a cigarette binds another red cell to this gas.

The long-term effects of this is what makes carbon monoxide so dangerous. The body cannot tolerate a reduced oxygen delivery so some secondary effects start to occur. A compensation for this lack of oxygen has to be arranged. An alarm system is triggered off to the bone marrow, where red cells are made, with the notion that if there is not enough oxygen being carried, then more oxygen carriers must be made. In other words the body compensates by making more red cells. This happens in every single smoker who has smoked for more than three months. This compensation sounds fine, but unfortunately those new red cells that have just been manufactured also travel to the lung and they too are exposed to the carbon monoxide and they too become bound up with it. The body does not know that there is a person behind this, wilfully smoking and inhaling carbon monoxide on a regular (about 200 times a day) basis! A third of the body's red cells bound up with carbon monoxide may be a fatal dose. Regular smokers have about a tenth of their red cells bound up. This is not a fatal dose but is certainly low grade carbon monoxide poisoning. The effect of increasing the red cell numbers over this period is that the circulation becomes sluggish. The red cells are not only not delivering the oxygen but there are too many of them. The carbon monoxide affects the clotability too. Too many sticky red cells packed together in the arteries are very deleterious to the circulation. It is evident in the areas of the circulation where the vessels are small, like the skin, the eyes, the brain and the heart. These are the areas where blood clots are most likely to occur.

All the effects of carbon monoxide are even worse for women. We know that women on the pill or any hormone replacement therapy worsens the clotting story. This is why women who smoke may have cold hands, cold feet and varicose veins, and why women on the pill are more likely to have clots. Smoking is a contra-indication for taking the pill.

What happens when you quit? What happens when no carbon monoxide enters the lung? The *very day* you do not smoke, the next newly made red cell that comes to the lung to do its job does not encounter any carbon monoxide and carries out its normal function. When enough of these cells start to deliver oxygen then the compensatory mechanism that has been in place, sometimes for decades, starts to wind down and less red cells are made. The effect is a thinning of the blood. This happens in every single smoker and takes altogether about four months to be completed. Every single cigarette you smoke after you've quit sets this process backwards.

It must be added here that *anything* that is smoked produces carbon monoxide. Marijuana creates large amounts of this gas. This also occurs with any 'roll your own cigarette'. The blood level of carbon monoxide from these types of cigarettes are higher not lower than manufactured cigarettes. Thus they are much worse for you.

Tar

Tar is a mixture of about a thousand different chemicals that have congealed together after burning as a glug of black sticky goo. It is called tar as it looks like that tar that is used to seal roads. This goo does not pass into the bloodstream as it is too heavy and thick. It depends on where that goo lands as to what happens to it, how it is destroyed and how it is got rid of. Smokers think that this tar is left lying around in the lung and simply accumulates over the years. If this was true smokers would fill up with tar and drown very soon after they had started smoking. Obviously this is not what happens. The tar is almost all destroyed and expelled from the body within a short period of time.

If tar lands on the upper part of the lung it is transported by the tiny hairy cells that only line that part of the lungs, called cilia. This cilia acts by wafting together and moving particles that are lying on top of it. The wafting movement in this case is upwards towards the mouth and the tar lying on top of the cilia is moved up over a period of about twelve hours. Unfortunately the cilia are also affected by nicotine. They are not as efficient as they should be and often waft out of sequence with each other. When the tar finally does get to the top of the lungs it is either coughed out or, more commonly, swallowed. You do not notice or feel the movement of cilia, but they move 24 hours a day. You may also not notice that you swallow the tar, which is then eliminated through the bowels. If the tar lands deep down in the lungs where there are no cilia, then most of that tar is destroyed by cells that are called macrophages. These cells surround the tar and literally gobble them up and take them away. The tar is destroyed over a period of about 24 hours.

Of course the old tar that has been taken away either by the cilia or by the macrophages is constantly being replaced with new tar and particles if you smoke regularly. A great deal of energy is put into this cleaning-up process. Ocassionally little clumps of tar are incorporated into the walls of the lung and unfortunately remain there. This is why you can always pick a smoker's lung by looking at it.

What happens, then, when someone stops smoking? The tar is simply not replaced and the lungs are cleared of most of it in a few days. No longer than that.

The inhalation of tobacco smoke may cause a constricting reaction in any part of the airways. This is due to the direct irritating effect of the particles deep inside the airways. But a smoker can often feel the clearing of the lung within a few days of quitting. Air flows quietly through your lungs and you may feel a lot less puffed going up and down the staircase.

Having described that the elimination of the most

important substances inhaled from smoking does not take very long, it's important to realise that this does not mean that there are no lasting effects from these chemicals even though they are no longer in the body. The effect for example on the wear and tear on the artery walls from expanding and contracting with nicotine remains. The constant effect of cleaning the lungs also puts excess wear and tear on the lining of the lung, causing areas of irritation and inflammation. The longer this has been going on the more extensive the wearing has become.

Nicotine and the heart

Besides being the main reason people smoke and being responsible for the addiction to smoking, nicotine has many unwanted side effects. Just as within seconds of inhaling the nicotine has gone to the brain cells that are craving, that same nicotine has as quick an effect on arteries. The nicotine causes the release of adrenalin, another neurotransmitter, which causes the muscles around arteries to constrict. When this happens the immediate reaction is a rise in blood pressure and heart rate. In fact if your blood pressure is measured while you smoke you can see the immediate rise; and then as the nicotine drops over the following half an hour so does your blood pressure. You can measure your own pulse rate changes too. Blood pressure and heart rate go up and down along with nicotine. There are even cases of patients having angina pectoris (acute chest pain) while smoking a cigarette.

However, we know that nicotine is very quickly broken down by the body. Within hours of smoking there is very little remaining. The liver and kidneys have begun to destroy it and it is metabolised, that is, pulled apart to its basic elements. The main metabolite is cotinine, which is an ineffectual, inactive substance that eventually passes out through the urine after about 36 hours. This means that within a day of having a cigarette nicotine can no longer have any effects as it is simply no longer there. The effects of a rise in blood pressure and a constriction of the blood vessels are also no longer there so that once there is no more active nicotine placed in the bloodstream the rise in blood pressure no longer occurs. The effect is immediate. The impact on the heart is also immediate.

Coronary artery disease

It has been postulated that the wear and tear on the arteries due to smoking, with the combined effect of carbon monoxide, are the major reasons that smokers are liable to suffer from this disease. Carbon monoxide impairs the carriage of oxygen to the myocardium, the heart muscle, so smoking sets a prime environment for those in the age group susceptible to heart attacks or myocardial infarction. But some of the effects of smoking appear to be reversible within days or weeks of quitting. Altogether the risk of having a heart attack is reduced by half after one year of not smoking.

Peripheral vascular disease

This is the disease of the arteries and veins ouside the heart. In smoking it is mainly caused by the combined effects of nicotine and carbon monoxide. This disease probably enjoys the most dramatic effect from quitting. On quitting, those suffering from arterial occlusions can look forward to a greatly increased ability to exercise and a reduced risk of amputation due to gangrene.

Emphysema, chronic bronchitis and asthma

The lungs are very obviously the prime target for diseases

from smoking for they are the vehicle used to inhale the smoke. Not all lung diseases are linked with smoking, but almost all are exacerbated by it. Emphysema in particular is a disease that is so linked with smoking that, like lung cancer, it is rare to develop it never having smoked. It is a disease of the tiny air sacs that are the main breathing entities of the lungs. The air passages of the lungs look like a large tree hanging upside down. Instead of leaves there are what look like millions of bunches of grapes. Each grape is a hollow air sac, called an alveolus, and each twig is a tube that brings air to that air sac. There are four million air sacs, two million in each lung. The lining of these sacs are elastic enough to stretch open when you take a big breath in and recoil when you breath out.

Emphysema, simply put, is a disease of the elastic recoil. Air must flow back and forth through the tubes smoothly, filling and emptying them with every breath in and out. In emphysema, the air sacs overinflate, recoil poorly and overstretch. Too much air is trapped in the lungs. Why this happens in smoking is complicated. The airways become inflamed from smoking, this then causes irritation and poor passage of air in and out of the tubes leading to the air sacs, which then cannot empty well. The ultimate effect is that stale air is not emptied out, which may leave the smoker eventually very breathless. This effect is irreversible. Some people seem to be susceptible to this reaction, others are not. Any family history of bronchitis predisposes smokers to emphysema. Though the effect is irreversible it does not progress after quitting. In other words apart from the natural reduction in airway elasticity that occurs in everyone there is no greater deterioration when you quit smoking. An anecdote goes that one alveolar wall is knocked out with every cigarette smoked. You can make a quick calculation: so many cigarettes, so many air sacs.

Bronchitis and chronic bronchitis have also been closely linked with smoking in that the inflammatory process occurs but it happens higher up in the larger tubes, or airways. This causes poor flow of air back and forth too. There is often a larger production of secretions due to the inflammation, something that can often be heard as wheezing and rattling.

Asthma is a complex and still poorly understood disease. Because of the inflammation that can occur due to smoking, the asthmatic is extremely sensitive to this and is liable to what is called hyperreactivity. Over-reacting to this irritation, the muscles around the airways constrict and don't allow air to flow in and out. These events are transient and can be helped with medication.

On stopping smoking there are some dramatic changes that occur in all these diseases. Respiratory symptoms of cough, sputum, wheeziness and shortness of breath can disappear rapidly on quitting, even after twenty years of smoking.

Another effect of nicotine that is not well known is that it reduces the cough reflex. At the top of the lungs there is a powerfully enervated area called the carina. This area is well endowed with nerves so that large particles that may enter the lungs by accident will be instantly coughed out. Nicotine has the effect of partially anaesthetising the carina. This is why most smokers do not cough like mad every time they inhale from a cigarette. It is only nicotine that does this, for if a smoker inhales smoke from a barbecue for example they do cough.

Again as soon as you stop smoking the cough reflex returns and you may find that you now have a cough when you didn't have one before. This cough doesn't last long and is part of the clearance that takes place just after quitting.

Chest infections like influenza and pneumonia are also more common in smokers than in those that don't smoke. Quitters quickly become like non-smokers.

Lung and throat cancer: risks and causes

Lung cancer is the disease that smokers fear the most, and justifiably so. It has become epidemic in its proportions in the last few decades. Lung cancer was considered a rarity in women until twenty years ago, but now it is as common in women as it is in men. If one looks at lung cancer rates over the last few decades in men only they are growing even though the actual amount of men smoking is decreasing steadily. We know that there is a lag time between the commencement of smoking and the development of lung cancer. It is at least fifteen years. But if we look for example at Australia in the 1950s when more than half the adult male population was smoking, we could expect a large number of lung cancers in the 1970s. There were certainly a lot, but as the years have passed there are less and less smokers but more and more lung cancers. What is going on? We also know that the more cigarettes actually smoked the greater the likelihood of developing cancer. Heavy smokers have twenty times the risk of light smokers of developing lung cancer. The data implies that the cigarette itself has become far more dangerous to each smoker. What is it in cigarette smoke that may cause the lung cancer and that has become so much more dangerous lately?

To date there have been many theories on this subject and much research has been carried out, even on animals, to be able to pinpoint one sole substance that may be the agent, that is, the carcinogen.

Suspects

Polonium (a relative of plutonium) is a radioactive substance found on the lining of the lungs after smoking. It is well known that radioactivity can be a cause of abnormal cell growth, but whether polonium is the agent in tobacco smoke is still undetermined.

The filter is a suspicious cause. Though its purpose is to filter some of the tar, it is made of small fibrous filaments that could easily be inhaled, and be the genesis of abnormal cells growing around it, not unlike asbestos fibres. It is said that 30,000 filters enter Sydney Harbour every day unbiodegraded.

Nicotine itself may be a culpable agent. Nicotine burned at very high temperatures can form nicotine nitrosamines, which are virulent carcinogens. Fascinating work carried out by Professor Dietrich Hoffman from the US Cancer Institute has shown that these nitrosamines cause organ-specific cancers. The specific organ he found was the lung.

Food colouring and flavouring. These are chemicals added to cigarette, cigar and pipe tobacco during their manufacturing. They are added to enhance the taste of the tobacco inhaled. However, when these substances are burned, many thousands of chemicals are emitted and little is known of their effect.

There are so many chemicals generated from smoking tobacco it's impossible to list them all here. What their separate or combined effects are is unknown. For example, saltpeter is added to the tobacco to help it burn and then it's inhaled by the smoker. Mentholated cigarettes have menthol added to them, almost all forms of pipe tobacco have sugars and flavourings added. What effects these have on the body is unknown.

Alcohol and tobacco products. Studies have shown that the combination of chronic alcohol and tobacco consumption greatly increases the risk of cancers of the oral cavity, oesophagus and larynx.

Other minor chemicals in tobacco smoke that may play a role in carcinogenesis are nickel, cadmium and arsenic.

Other cancers
Lung cancer is the most prominent cancer implicated with smoking but there are others such as oesophageal, bladder and kidney cancers.

Ulcers: peptic, gastric and duodenal
Probably the cause of these ulcers is the increase of gastric secretion that occurs with smoking. There is an increase in the acidity of these secretions and more reflux occurs. Most of the mechanisms that cause these ulcers seem to be rapidly reversible on stopping smoking. Again there is a dose relationship in the healing process: the fewer cigarettes smoked, the greater the healing. The irony is that medication taken for hypersecretion is almost completely negated by smoking.

Curious medical benefits from stopping
There are some other positive health effects of quitting that are not very well known to the community.

🚭 In women, menopause comes on several years earlier if you smoke but is normal if you quit.

🚭 In men, there is evidence that sperm density is reduced in smokers and returns to normal on quitting. Penile erection is also affected by smoking through reduced blood flow to the penis, but returns to normal on cessation.

🚬 Blood cholesterol levels drop in every smoker when they quit smoking, even if the diet has not changed.

🚬 Smokers report more days off work due to illness and injury than non-smokers.

🚬 Many opthalmologists swear that they can pick a smoker from a non-smoker when they look into their eyes. The very tiny vessels on the back of the eye are clogged up with blood, a 'sausage-like' effect, and this disappears within a few months of smoking. This may be why some smokers feel they can see better when they've quit.

🚬 Wounds and scratches heal faster when you no longer smoke.

Unlike alcohol abuse, to date there is no evidence that an ex-smoker has any residual brain cell damage. This is important as the effects of nicotine act directly on the neuron and could affect the structure of these cells, permanently affecting brain function.

Some non-clinical benefits of quitting

Wrinkling. This effect from smoking has been hard to measure. The aptly named 'dog's bottom' is a phenomenon well noticed around women's mouths who smoke. Whether this is caused by constant pursing of the lips around a cigarette or by poorer blood suppy to the skin is not well understood. 'Crow's feet' at the corners of the eyes have also been noted. Certainly there is anecdotal evidence that the skin is fresher and healthier on quitting, which is probably due to better oxygenation.

Sense of smell and taste. The 'return' of these two senses often has interesting effects. Smokers are often horrified to realise that smoking smells so badly but their sense of smell is also stronger for pungent odours like the garbage bin, which they may have hardly smelled before. Food tastes a great deal stronger now that flavours are much more discernible. This may be linked with an increased appetite but is probably not.

Smoking and occupation

It's extraordinary that many occupations that involve the inhalation of dust and chemicals have had health and safety regulations for decades that are justly severe in protecting the worker, but a key element to the potential for disease and death was ignored. To better illustrate this, for example, those working in the asbestos industry have had strict regulations covering their handling and working with this substance. However, the calculated mortality ratios from cancer (the ratio of death in smokers versus never smokers) is 87 in smokers working with asbestos compared to five in non-smokers working with asbestos. That means more than fifteen times the risk of getting lung cancer just because you smoke! The same risks occur in other mining industries as well.

Women's health in smoking cessation

There has been a misconception in the past that women were somehow immune from heart attacks, vascular disease and cancers. Fortunately it is now clear in the minds of most individuals that women can experience the same consequences as men if they smoke, and more. There are particular diseases that occur only to women and these are also increasing along with the rise in smoking in women. Along with the rise in lung cancers, cervical and breast cancers have now been linked to cigarette smoking. Problems rise dramatically with women who are pregnant. The foetus and newborn baby are more susceptible to abnormalities and low birth-weight, and the mother is more likely to suffer complications during pregnancy.

We know that:

🚭 Smoking and oral contraception, the pill, greatly increase the risk of cerebral subarachnoid haemorrhage.

🚭 Women who stop smoking before they become pregnant have children with birthweights the same as women who have never smoked.

🚭 Quitting in the first three months and remaining abstinent for the rest of the pregnancy protects the foetus from the effects of smoking.

🚭 Women who cut down but do not quit *do not* protect the foetus.

🚭 Fertility is much reduced by smoking.

Passive smoking and health risk factors

This book is devoted to the smoker trying to quit and not to berating smokers. However, an aspect of passive smoking that is important in the issue of quitting is passive nicotine and passive carbon monoxide, and the effect these have on the children of smokers and quitters.

Passive nicotine

We now know that addicted smokers have a reaction to nicotine that other people do not have. They can become sensitive to this nicotine in that inhaling it may trigger off a neurological reaction. This continues to occur well after they have quit and necessary precautions need to be made. For the ex-smoker avoidance is the key.

What about the passive never-smoker? There is a legitimate concern that young children who are passive smokers may become reactive to the nicotine they inhale. This is especially worrying as the latest evidence shows that the addiction may be hereditary. We can certainly measure nicotine in the bloodstream of toddlers whose parents smoke, even in newborn babies who are breast-fed by mothers who smoke. These children are unable to take the option of leaving the room, and run the risk of becoming dependent on the most addictive substance known to humankind way before they can even speak let alone buy a packet of cigarettes at the supermarket.

Passive carbon monoxide

In the new ex-smoker as well as the never-smoker inhaling from someone else's cigarette includes inhaling the carbon monoxide produced. Though it is diluted by the room or environment you are standing in, this carbon monoxide has exactly the same effects as mentioned before. Some passive smokers may be working in small confined spaces that have little ventilation. We studied the carbon monoxide levels of a non-smoking barman. He worked in a very smoky environment. By the end of a night's shift he would have the same levels of carbon monoxide as an active twenty-a-day smoker; he was effectively a smoker who did not smoke. For him, as with others like him, he suffers the medical consequences of being a smoker. He has the same risks of heart disease and lung cancer as an active smoker.

Enough evidence has been gathered to show that someone living with a smoker is at risk of developing lung cancer and heart disease. In both these diseases, the more cigarettes the smoker smokes, the greater the risk the other person has. This dose-relationship is the clincher in the evidence on passive smoking.

Most horrifying to the parents of asthmatic children is that their smoking has a direct effect on their children's asthma. Many studies have shown that these children have much less frequent asthma attacks when their parents quit smoking, especially if the mother was a smoker. This is because the mother is usually more often around the child than the father. Even non-asthmatic children have higher likelihood of coughs, colds and flus if their parents are smokers.

The beneficial effects of nicotine

Nicotine as we know causes many fatal diseases. It cannot be discounted that there is evidence that nicotine may hep in resisting the acquistion of some unusual diseases. Statistical analysis has shown that smokers are less likely to get Alzheimer's disease, Parkinson's disease and Tourette's syndrome. These are all diseases of the nervous system and it can easily be imagined that nicotine may play a role in diminishing the likelihood of acquiring them. Nicotine, in forms other than smoking, has been positively used in research as therapy for some of the symptoms of these diseases. Two other diseases unrelated to each other are also diseases of non-smokers and have also been treated with nicotine. They are ulcerative colitis and aphthous stomatitis. These are all factual curiosities which show that there may be a therapeutic value for nicotine. It is important to note, however, *there has never been a therapeutic value found for smoking tobacco.*

🚭 7 🚭

The learning experience of quitting

It is said that most smokers, addicted or not, need to have several attempts to quit before they quit for good. The evidence for this has not been very well tested but certainly looks real. Smokers attending a clinic have reported at least two attempts to quit before going to specialists for help. Some smokers find it increasingly more difficult with each attempt, while others find it is the same every time. There is no evidence that the older you get the harder it gets, but some individuals feel that this is true for them. Certainly every attempt to quit should be a learning experience for you, and can easily be a positive one, though it may not be obvious at the time. You can learn how to avoid the traps that occurred. Focus on the event. What were the bad things that happened? What were the good things that happened? How can you avoid the bad and enhance the good?

If you have made it several days or even weeks you certainly will be aware that the thoughts about smoking diminish. This is a positive result; the going away of symptoms of withdrawal. Many smokers believe they will have cravings and discomfort forever. Desperately missing cigarettes every day of their lives. If this was the case nobody would have ever been able to quit, they would all have eventually succumbed to the need to smoke. Imagine having cravings every day and *not* giving in? This doesn't happen. But what if you did have very serious cravings that overwhelmed you within the first days you tried? Then obviously your dependency is quite severe and you may need extra help in a clinic that specialises in this. The recognition that this is a real problem is slowly entering the medical profession and many physicians are taking a real interest in this problem. If your physician still thinks you need to go it alone, seek advice elsewhere.

> MENTHOL CIGARETTES DO NOT COME FROM MENTHOLATED TOBACCO LEAVES. THE MENTHOL IS ADDED DURING PRODUCTION.

There are some experts in the United States and in Great Britain who believe there are smokers who, given that tobacco is accessible, will never be able to quit. They believe that the withdrawals in these people are so severe no amount of treatment will be able to support them. There are certainly cases that look particularly grim, but they are very rare. Each and every person entering a clinic believes they are the worst case ever seen. This is definitely not so. Do not use this excuse to never attempt to quit again. Even though each smoker is an individual the basic problem is the same for each; it is the degree that is different. If the main problems that have concerned you have been loneliness and boredom or an inability to cope with stress or depression then a committed effort to do something about these issues can result in a positive outcome. All types of alternatives to smoking are available to cope with these life problems from an enhancement of your social life to an exercise regime.

A multitude of combined forces influence individuals to contemplate quitting. There may be social pressures, family pressures, health reasons, ideas on self-control, ideas on self-indulgence and influences from the anti-smoking campaigns. Whatever they are, the basic ability to take control of your own life seems to be a strong and pertinent element. The ability to affect an outcome and the learning of coping skills also have a bearing on the decision to quit. When smokers throw up their hands and say 'I can't do anything about this' they may mean 'I have no control over my destiny'. Taking a positive viewpoint on the future has been implicit in the wish to quit smoking and stay quit, irrespective of whether the quitting is difficult or not, the dependency is high or low.

These are some case studies that show relatively typical reactions some people show when they try to quit, or their ideas about quitting. You may see yourself in some of these people, and be helped by their experiences.

Yannis: he needed a heart attack

Yannis, better known as John today, came from Greece twenty years ago. In the village where he came from everyone smoked. It was unheard of for a man not to smoke! When he arrived in Australia, many men were smoking here too. He felt at home with it, though the drinking of beer was something that was foreign to him. Every day he woke to a thick black coffee and a dark Turkish cigarette. He worked at the fish markets where he could smoke freely and he and his friends would take breaks together over a cigarette. The notion of his own health and well-being was culturally foreign to John. He had no idea about fitness, blood cholesterol levels or anything remotely linked to a healthy lifestyle.

As John grew older, it was his children that impressed him with the idea that smoking was something he should stop doing. They had begun to learn at school of the physical harm that smoking was doing, not only to their father's health but also to their own. John spent a great deal of time in the beginning arguing with the kids. Hadn't Grandfather Michaelis smoked and lived to 90? The kids argued back that Grandfather was an exception and that there were others that got sickly and others again that had died.

Yannis denied the evidence put before him for a long time. This was a good life and all this stuff about smoking was stupid. When he did make a half-hearted attempt to not smoke, he let fly with a terrible temper. Everyone in the family made a secret wish that he would smoke again. He too was relieved when his friends came around at the end of the day and dragged him off to his favourite coffee shop, where they could laugh it off over a cigarette.

But something occurred that changed his mind radically. One day he had chest pains that overwhelmed him. They wouldn't go away. John agreed to let a doctor come, something that was rare for him. His life floated by him. He saw his wife in black, crossing herself. When he had recovered well enough from this heart attack he began to have discussions with his doctor and an agreement was made between them that John should seriously quit smoking. His doctor explained to him that he was addicted to nicotine. He had trouble believing this because the notion of being an addict, like a heroin addict, was ridiculous to him. Nonetheless he agreed to test himself out. John started using Nicorette. He complained because he never chewed chewing gum.

(This was good because he wasn't supposed to chew them.) John was surprised that he could spend a great deal of the day using the Nicorette and not get angry or nervous with the people around him.

It was the hardest for him not to smoke with his coffee. When his friends came around and they all smoked and laughed at him it got quite tough. He learned to say to his pals that it was doctor's orders that he shouldn't smoke. That was a well-respected solution and accepted by everyone, though begrudgingly. It had become so much part of the ritual of his life, so automatic. Every time he felt like a cigarette he got a notion into his head that this whole smoking thing was a matter of pride in the end and he was not going to let it get to him. Life was more important than anything else. This helped him a great deal. Even though inside himself there were sometimes strong urges to smoke and he felt less of a man because he was not smoking, especially in front of his friends, he doggedly pursued not smoking.

As the days passed he became more and more resigned to it and slowly, over time, stopped thinking about cigarettes most of the time. He even stopped using the Nicorettes after a few months. He had lost interest in it. Now and again he was, to be honest, gripped with nostalgia for a cigarette, but in the end he rationalised that not smoking was saving his life. The picture of his wife crossing herself said it all to him; he used it as a logo every time it occurred to him to smoke.

Mary: the drinker

Mary had been smoking since she was a teenager. She smoked at school behind the sheds, or in the toilets. She thought then that it was a bit of fun, a bit scandalous and definitely grown up. Her parents were infuriated even though they themselves smoked. Mary became more and more involved with smoking as she grew older, smoking all the way through her pregnancies, including a miscarriage. Occasionally Mary thought she should stop smoking, especially after a night of partying and drinking. Her hangovers were pretty ghastly. Not until she was turning forty did it occur to her that in the end her smoking was making her look old. None of her friends smoked any more. She was feeling more and more like an outsider, a leper. At work she had to sneak around to have a cigarette, not unlike her school days.

Mary's level of dependency was not as great as she thought it might be. She had simple changes to make in her behaviour that would help her along. She resigned herself not to drink any alcohol for at least a month because she realised the influence it had over her smoking. A break from drinking would do her good but she was terrified that she would put on weight, convinced that everyone did when they quit. Her friends were very supportive, taking her off to play a game of tennis or go for a swim when she looked like weakening.

After four days of being pretty crabby and chewing a lot of peppermints, she secretly decided to find the cigarettes she had hidden away from everyone's prying eyes. It wasn't as if she had an overwhelming urge to smoke just then, but she felt as if she wanted a treat, a reward for not having smoked. She had a secret cigarette in the garage. It didn't even taste good to her, it made her head spin. She left disgusted and demoralised.

Smoking that one cigarette had two effects on Mary. First, she got depressed about the fact that she had no control over herself. She thought to herself that having had that one had broken the 'spell' and that she may as well go on smoking now. The second effect that she was not aware of was that nicotine had entered her bloodstream again and started off a cascade of chemical reactions. Even though she thought she could restrict herself to a couple a day, these two reactions had Mary back to smoking regularly within days.

A couple of weeks later it occurred to Mary that she might try it again, having understood the pitfalls from the last attempt. This time she held out. She was aware that as time passed things got better, not worse. She was able to smell cigarette smoke on other people's clothes for the first time. It disgusted her that she must have smelt like that. Her winter clothes particularly smelled bad, so she got out a jumper every time she felt like a cigarette and put her nose into it. Everyone commented on her looks. She looked well and fresh, because she was a lot less tired. Her biggest concern was what would happen if there was some catastrophe or other. How would she react?

Soon she became indifferent to other people smoking around her, in fact she rather hated it and was the first one to move away from smokers at a restaurant. But most surprising of all was the strange effect she now got from alcohol. She couldn't 'hold' her drinks as she once did. One glass of wine was like two or three before. She really had to be careful how much she drank now. She also realised that 'the morning after the night before' was due to her smoking and not so much to her drinking. Most important of all was the fact that she did not put on weight, mostly because she wasn't drinking so much. Mary never counted on that!

Peter: the aggressor
Peter is an accountant. He is meticulous in everything he does. He has been smoking only since his late twenties. He is now thirty-five. Since he started smoking he has always wished he could stop. He started smoking when he married because his wife smoked. She quit easily

when she got pregnant but he kept on. He knows all the physical effects of smoking, but gets agitated and can't concentrate on his work without them. He is his own boss, so smoking is not an issue at the office. His secretary also smokes, though they make a point not to smoke in front of clients. His secretary has often had to hold on to his cigarettes for him. His instructions to her are 'Only give them to me if I'm desperate.' She has often refused him a cigarette, but in the end had to give in.

Peter has often tried solutions to stop smoking. He went along to a hypnotherapist. On leaving the clinic he felt a strange relief, felt good and didn't feel like a cigarette. He felt good for about a day but then began to get anxious and agitated; he felt as if it had worn off. He also got very aggressive with his clients. This actually frightened Peter because it was very unlike him. He was soon back at his secretary's desk begging for a cigarette. He heard about a new technology in medicine called transdermal nicotine patches. He went along to his doctor and they discussed his smoking problem. He scored a 7 on the dependency scale.

Peter got a packet of nicotine patches and started using them that night. His first sensation was that he really didn't have a desire to smoke, none at all. It had vanished. He couldn't help but be sceptical, being an accountant. But each day was like the next. He was simply not interested in smoking. The only strange reaction he had was that he had the weirdest dreams. His doctor assured him this was normal. After a while the dreams ceased to occur. According to the instructions he reduced the concentration of patches after several weeks of each. Though they were pretty expensive Peter calculated the savings he would have over the years, and figured it was worth it. What surprised Peter most of all was how simple it had been.

He has never looked back. He is now fascinated by why he was smoking and the addictiveness of it. He has learned every single aspect of smoking and its effects. He is adamant that he will never smoke again.

Tracey: the socialite

Tracey is young. She's 22 and very happy-go-lucky. Tracey lives the good life, and has a terrific social circle that includes many friends. She smokes about fifteen cigarettes a day, but that can treble when she's out at night, and she's out a lot. All her girlfriends smoke. Every time she has gone along to her doctor for a renewal for her prescription of the pill her doctor warns her that she shouldn't be smoking and taking the pill at the same time. She shrugs this off.

Her boyfriend hates her smoking. She pretends that this doesn't bother her too much either. She has had an ambivalence about smoking. On the one hand she hates the idea that smoking will be physically detrimental to her in the future, but on the other she can't seem to socialise without it. She couldn't possibly give up her social life, her friends and her drinking after all. Smoking gives her confidence. She feels she needs a cigarette to express herself, to occupy her hands and to hide behind when she feels embarrassed.

When Tracey makes efforts not to smoke, usually to cut down, it is usually short lived. She can manage to go to her aunty's place, where it is strictly not on, and not smoke for two weeks but it's virtually impossible to get away from the influences she has back at home and at work.

She will need a great deal of 'change of attitude" before she will be ready to quit. Her social life is more important to her than her well-being. In her case she is simply not able to cope with the peer-group pressure and cues that surrounds her, though she would be mortified if she understood that this is what she was influenced by. She goes with the flow. It will take some maturing for Tracey to quit permanently.

Terry: the marijuana smoker

Terry is the type of smoker that can take it or leave it. He is a photographer, fairly free living, and sees himself as particularly artistic. Terry smokes a lot of marijuana, at least a joint a day. For him this substance enhances his creativity and heightens his sensitivity to the world around him. He mixes it with tobacco to reduce the harshness of the straight marijuana, and to dilute it so that it's not so expensive. The fact that cigarette smoking has become so socially difficult for Terry (he can't smoke in his favourite Paddington restaurant) has made him decide to quit.

However, Terry gets caught in the trap of having the joint and then needing a cigarette. He notices that the need to smoke cigarettes is bound up with the need to use marijuana. Terry has heard that smoking this amount of marijuana is not harmful to his health nor is it addictive, so why give it up? The fact that Terry is using an illegal substance is of no relevance to him whatsoever. As many times as he attempts to stop smoking cigarettes he continues to because of the marijuana trap. Terry will have to learn to stop smoking anything at all, to get away from the connotation of holding a cigarette-like item in his hand. If he doesn't stop smoking marijuana he will not stop smoking cigarettes.

Joyce: hooked on Nicorette

Joyce was a smoker for many years and has quit successfully using the Nicorette gum. This was almost a year ago and Joyce has never really had any problems with not smoking. She has been able to work and socialise without any difficulties, escept that lately she's became embarrassed by the chewing. She didn't like getting out a gum in public and felt that there were prying eyes, ready to judge her as 'addicted to the gum'. Even Joyce's chemist didn't like selling them to her any more. He complained that he wouldn't keep on suppling them to her for much longer, and that she should make an effort to stop using them. She too really believed that she was hooked on the gum.

Joyce made a phone call one day to her local Smokers' Clinic, who gaver her some very useful tips. She was to cut the gums in half and every day substitute one whole gum for a half a gum. She did this slowly over ten days. She was then told to substitute the half Nicorettes with any other non-sweet gum she could find. She did this over the next ten days. She did have the occasional yearn for a real Nicorette, but a month later Joyce realised that she was no longer interested in chewing anything at all, and simply dropped it.

What had happened to Joyce was not unusual: she was not hooked on the Nicorette but still hooked on nicotine. When she started to reduce the amount of nicotine by halving the doses and then diluting it with other gums she was able to wean herself off the Nicorettes without any difficulty.

Joe: the taxi driver

Joe, who is 50, has been a taxi driver for ten years. In these ten years Joe estimates that he has smoked millions of cigarettes. He must smoke 50 a shift, he figures, at least! He smokes particularly more when on shifts in the early morning. He is so bored he stands at the cab rank waiting for a fare and just smokes one after the other.

Joe's situation changed somewhat when smoking was

banned in taxis, but he still managed to smoke a lot when there were no customers, and always smoked along with customers that smoked in the cab. He often broke the rules and only threw the cigarettes out if the customers complained. He says that he smokes because he's bored and nervous. Financially, he has trouble making ends meet. Business is terrible and he only just keeps his act together. He swears he doesn't enjoy smoking at all, he hates it. His wife gets pretty angry with him, because not only is his smoking messy but he's always burning holes in his clothes. Joe would never admit to her how many times he's nearly had an accident when he's dropped a lit cigarette in his lap while driving.

One day Joe drove a patient to a smoker's clinic in the city. 'Does this do any good?' asked Joe. The customer was really keen and told Joe he couldn't have quit without the support and counselling he got in there. Joe thought, 'This is providence.' He went in then and there to enrol before he got cold feet. For a few days he was to keep a strict record of his smoking: of each cigarette, and when and where he did it. He said this would be too cumbersome in the cab, but he was told that if he could light a cigarette while driving he could note it down on a pad without too much trouble.

Just keeping note of what he was doing cut Joe's smoking down to the essential cigarettes. He wasn't even trying and counted 30 a day instead of his usual 50 plus. He returned with this account to the clinic, where the counsellor pointed out that the time intervals between his cigarettes were not arbitrary but very regular, about every 40 minutes. He was told about his addiction and that it was categorised as severe. He scored 10 in the Fagerström scale. He was prescribed the 4 mg Nicorette gum and he was to commence the next day when he got up. He was encouraged to use it as often as he thought about a cigarette. He found that it tasted pretty terrible and gave him heartburn, but found that he was smoking now about five or six cigarettes a day.

When he reported to the clinic they were pleased but not pleased enough to leave him smoking six a day. Joe thought it was pretty good to get down to that number in a couple of days, but the counsellor insisted that it was out, not down. Joe agreed not to chew the gum so vigorously, which is what gave him the heartburn, and he got used to the taste of the gum after a while. He found with the techniques he was taught at the clinic and the reporting in that he regularly had to do that not smoking began to wear on him. It was not too difficult after all. He got so used to the gum that once he said to a friend without thinking twice that he 'smoked about fifteen Nicorettes a day'. He was worried that there would be a need to use the gum indefinitely, but he was assured that the need to use the gum would go down with time, and so it did. He was surprised mostly with the fact that he did not miss it that much, that the activity itself was not that important.

He looked at the other cabbies at the rank to get clues as to what the non-smokers were doing when they were waiting for a fare. They had exactly the same problems as he did, business was as bad for them as it was for him. They didn't resort to smoking or drinking to deal with it, nor did he. He leaned to stroll around, take in the fresh air, read more, do crosswords to pass the time. He too was saving money not smoking. When he got down to about eight gums a day he was advised to swap to the 2 mg Nicorette, which he did. He did that with no trouble but found that he was using about fifteen of them a day. He was told not to be concerned, that it would diminish in time. Joe attended the clinic for three months and became very attached to the staff there.

He no longer chews Nicorette but is always worried at the back of his mind that if there was a crisis he might resort to a cigarette again.

Mike: an AIDS victim

Mike, 35, was diagnosed HIV positive two years ago. Until then Mike lived an extraordinarily active social life. He drank, smoked and ate anything he liked. Since diagnosis nearly all of this has changed. Mike eats the right foods, is very conscientious about exercising regularly and drinks in moderation. He even ensures that he gets a good amount of sleep instead of burning the candle at both ends as he used to do. His only bug is smoking. He can't seem to get a grip on staying off it.

In his mind Mike fluctuates between the wish to quit and the inevitability of his death. 'What's the point? It's too late.' Mike floats in this ambivalence only in his smoking. In controlling his diet, the alcohol and even sex he has no real problem, but smoking holds a special part in his person that is different from the others. It is his friend, his comfort. His ernest attempts to quit come to a grinding halt after about three or four days. That Mike might be addicted to nicotine doesn't enter his head, and if it did, or if it was pointed out to him, the problems would remain the same, as Mike has yet to be convinced that he will be better off without smoking. Until Mike understands this he will not quit, and then it may be too late.

Russell: the asthmatic

Russell was in his fifties and had had asthma for at least twenty years. He knew what brought it on: spring, drinking beer, laughing a lot and smoking too much. Russell's doctor had told him a thousand times to stop smoking or he would eventually develop emphysema, but again,

Russell couldn't see the point in quitting as he felt 'the damage was done'. His wife and children were adamant that he should do something too, but they more or less left him alone with it because after all it was his choice. Russell's asthma was definitely getting worse over the years as he got older. He coudn't go running up the stairs as before but often had to stop and hold on to the railing and catch his breath on the way up. He was prescribed some cortisone to inhale for each spring season along with his puffer.

One night after a long day of smoking more than usual Russell woke with an increasingly irritating cough. As he coughed he got wheezier but he found his puffer didn't seem to do much good. That night he got so distressed and breathless that his wife dressed him and took him to the casualty section of the hospital. Russell could hardly breathe all the way there. He opened the car window to get some air. A packet of his cigarettes was lying on the front seat of the car. Russell threw them out the window. He got to the hospital and was given a strong nebuliser and in the morning was sent home.

Russell has not had a cigarette since. In the beginning, after the initial shock wore off he had the occasional longing for a cigarette but now he is not even interested. His asthma has improved dramatically, he rarely needs any medication and he gets to the top of the stairs, not running, but not puffed either.

Sue: the exerciser
Sue is in her thirties, an executive in a computer company. She is busy but sets time aside three times a week to go to the gym, where she is a member. She wouldn't miss out on this, and feels deprived when she can't exercise. She is fit and well. But she smokes about a packet a day. In the scoring mechanism she rates a 7.

She smokes about 25 a day spread evenly over the day. She rarely drinks, watches her diet and generally has a quiet but sociable life. Sue justifies her smoking because she feels it relaxes her. She has coffee breaks with a cigarette, and after work she has a few cigarettes when she gets home after a hard day. As far as she is concerned her exercising negates all the ill effects from smoking, which she knows all about.

There is no convincing Sue that this is otherwise. Even her gym instructor tells her that she would improve her fitness if she quit smoking, but since Sue can exercise at levels far higher than most of the others in her class, she hardly feels that it's relevant to her, considering that she is so fit. In Sue's case little will change until she either becomes aware that she is addicted to cigarettes, she develops a medical complication from it or she notices that she is aging faster than normal. It may take decades before she herself inevitably realises that something should be done about her smoking.

Some of these examples have had a medical event that triggered off a dramatic change in their thoughts towards smoking; some have had a slow change that has taken years to accomplish. Some have been successful quitters and others have not. It would be at an enormous health cost though, if we had to wait for every nicotine addict to have a medical problem before they decided to quit. To never reach this point should be the strategy most smokers should take.

🚭 **8** 🚭

Maintaining the rage

The last thing an ex-smoker wants to become is a rabid anti-smoking convert. Most smokers shudder at this idea but it is not uncommon to find recent quitters zealously trying to talk all their smoking friends into quitting. Sometimes individuals need to 'hang their hat' on some focal point so as to be able to concentrate their energies on never smoking again. Some new quitters throw themselves into a regime of physical fitness and others collect information and pamphlets on smoking to distribute around the workplace. Others bore their friends to tears with endless accounts of how they did it, as if they have discovered a new religion. Ideally none of this is to the advantage of a new quitter and wears thin on their friends and colleagues. A totally new you is unrealistic and ultimately impractical. How then do you maintain the idea of not smoking into the months ahead? How does the idea of a cigarette become a non-event? Will you become indifferent to the sight of a packet of your favourite brand of cigarettes in time? This is usually hard to believe, the idea that you may simply not be interested at all in smoking but, just as the daily need to smoke dissipated, so in time does the whole idea of smoking.

It is not uncommon to have moments of nostalgia about smoking. Most ex-smokers cope with this by shrugging it off, using various strategies from being relieved to deciding that if smoking was healthy they would do it again but since it is not there is no way they would consider starting to smoke again.

Here are some other items that can be used as a source of concentration and consternation should the need arise.

Logo therapy

This therapy was devised by Victor Frankl, whose own experiences helped him to devise strategies for people who were struggling with adversity. From his work has developed logo therapy, which is easily adapted to addictions and the combating of cravings and anxiety and moments of temptation. Simply put, Frankl recommends that you focus your attentions on the particular reason you want to stay stopped. You must picture this in your mind's eye. For example, if you wish never to smoke again because your lungs are in poor shape, then picture in your mind's eye yourself sitting up in the middle of the night coughing uncontrollably as you may often have done in the past. If you wish to stay stopped for your children, then place them in a cameo in your mind. Your 'logo' can be a jar of money, a relative or friend with cancer, whatever your main reason for quitting was. This is your logo. You should practice bringing this logo into your mind so that it becomes an automatic thought that you equate with smoking. Your logo can be brought into your thoughts when you feel temptations to smoke.

The politics of tobacco

Some ex-smokers use their newly acquired energies to

delve into the politics of tobacco. This is an area that many new quitters get very angry about. They feel that over the years they have been had. The industry has manipulated them as adolescents with advertising and that by being hooked the whole of their lives they have fallen into a trap. All of this is true. One of the general all-time nasties of this century must surely be the tobacco promoters. They have skilfully managed to make a product seem attractive to each individual. A man's cigarette, a woman's cigarette, the sporty cigarette, the elegant cigarette, the young woman's cigarette etc. (In the USA there is even a cigarette called 'Ebony' marketed to African-Americans.) Yet each one contains exactly the same substance.

Some new ex-smokers maintain their rage by booking non-smoking restaurants only so as not to be in areas of temptation. Others write to politicians or write letters to the editor when items about smoking occur in the press. This is a far more reasonable reaction and more likely to have an impact in helping protect others, particularly kids from being initiated into the addiction.

Kids as targets

Most smokers are not aware that for every smoker that quits (or dies) at least one new one must be recruited to keep sales steady. In Australia, for example, 20,000 smokers die each year, so at least 20,000 new ones must be found to replace them to keep sales equal. These new smokers are never adults 'changing brands' as claimed by the tobacco industry, but inevitably are kids buying into the smoking habit like all the smokers before them. Once they're in, they're usually on the conveyor belt for life until they fall off and are replaced by the next generation.

A recent survey in the USA showed that 30 per cent

of three year olds recognised a particular logo as a cigarette brand, and by six years of age 60 per cent recognised the brand! It is folly to believe that children are not influenced by this.

There is no reason why young people who smoke should not be as addicted as adults who smoke. The addiction does not take years to acquire, just as tolerance to the side effects of smoking does not take years. It seems that adolescents can have as difficult a time in quitting as adults. The difference is that many kids don't try to quit so they don't know they have a problem with it. It is only when they make an attempt to not smoke for a while that they notice their smoking is not a random controllable event. They are often under the impression that they can take it or leave it, and will often lie to their elders about this.

Rather than badger a young smoker about their future illness, which is as remote to them as the moon, a good ploy with an adolescent is to suggest to them that perhaps they are hooked. Most will vigorously deny this. Then suggest that if they are not hooked they should be able to go at least a week without a cigarette. Some might notice that they find this quite difficult. The whole concept of being addicted to cigarettes usually never occurs to them. The other concern, particularly of adults and teachers, is what to do about a child who smokes and is caught openly doing it. Most adults are distressed by this even if they themselves are smokers. Nothing is more ludicrous than an adult coming up to a school kid and telling them, 'Don't smoke, you'll regret it like I do.'

Studies have shown that if these children are given an open policy on their smoking they will use it liberally and are more likely to become full-on adult smokers. It's rather the 'give them a hand, they'll take your whole arm'.

However, if their smoking is very restricted, this means no smoking in the house, no special rooms set aside to smoke etc., these adolescents are less likely to become adult smokers. This may seem Draconian, but the evidence is that this seems to work in many cases. Of course it is implicit in the above discussion that kids have access to tobacco, which they undoubtedly have, though it is against the law not only to sell cigarettes to any person under the age of eighteen but to even 'provide' them with one.

Women as targets

With women being perceived as new consumers in the 1960s and 1970s they have been prime targets for

THE CONSEQUENCES OF SMOKING ARE FAR MORE SERIOUS THAN THE WEIGHT GAINED FROM QUITTING. TWO AND A HALF KILOS IS THE AVERAGE GAIN.

tobacco advertising. Many women were sucked into the glamour image that was sold to them. Today some women still fall for it, but in a different way. The roll-your-own, wear-it-in-your-belt package is targeted at the 'liberated woman'. These cigarettes have the image that they are somehow ecologically sounder than other brands. This must be so if you roll it yourself? The tobacco and paper is the same, but because they burn more freely more carbon monoxide is made, not less, and there is no filter to extract large particles, which is altogether much worse for the smoker. The great weight gain debate has fallen nicely into the hands of the tobacco industry. Nothing must be more gratifying for them than women equating smoking with slimness.

Tobacco would never have been so freely marketed

and sold had it come into existence in the second half of this century. However, history has made it legitimate, so we are generally stuck with the saleability of one of the most addictive substance known.

New markets
It also is now well known that as the markets diminish in the western world, the tobacco industries are seeking markets where there are susceptible individuals, where laws do not protect the consumer and where the health authorities have little power.

These areas are particularly Asia and Africa. There is even a race into the newer markets of Eastern Europe, where there is little regulation but large populations with money to spend. (It was recently reported that a cigarette brand was to be launched in Poland called 'Solidarity'.) More insidious than this is the fact that these less industrialised nations have poorer health facilities to deal with the medical repercussions of smoking. The general health and well-being of Africans is well below that of Europeans, for example. Therefore, smoking amongst Africans has far graver repercussions than it has on, say, Europeans.

As mentioned before, flavourings have always been added to the tobacco to make it more palatable. It was rumoured recently that in Brazil there will be new brands available with tropical fruit flavourings.

Growing tobacco
As mentioned previously, the contents of today's cigarettes is considered to be particularly lethal. However, there is little regulation accorded to the maufacturers as to what tobacco used for smoking contains. Most governments tacitly approve of the so-called self-regulatory codes.

Genetics of growing insect-resistant strains

A very doubtful aspect of the tobacco that is used for consumption today is their insect resistance. Most people know nothing about tobacco farming and are left relatively ignorant of the process that brings the leaf from the ground to the neatly packeted little cigarette in a box. Tobacco was always prone to blight, rust, insects and rot. Various chemical sprays were added to the leaves as they grew to prevent these illnesses. Today, however, with the advent of genetic engineering many plants can be made resistant to illnesses from the seed onwards. The idea that one is inhaling a substance whose DNA has been tampered with often horrifies smokers when they become aware of this.

Growth of tobacco in Africa and the tree scandal

One of the few unreported scandals of the 1970s and 1980s is the planting of tobacco in Africa. In Australia the government has reduced the tobacco quotas gradually so that the subsidies that supported the farmers are ceasing to exist. Our farmers have been encouraged to diversify to other industries. This has occurred in other progressive nations where tobacco is grown as well. However, since the growing of tobacco has become limited in the west, the large tobacco corporations have found that Malawi, Kenya, Tanzania and parts of Zimbabwe are good areas to grow tobacco and can give farmers access to a quick cash crop. Catch 22. To be able to sell their tobacco the farmers must bail it dried or it will rot. It is the job of the tobacco farmer to dry the leaves. In Africa, drying leaves seems to be simple enough. Place the leaves out on racks and let it be sun dried.

Unfortunately this is not quick enough so the farmers have been encouraged to build kilns to dry the leaves using wood fires. Where does the wood come from? Since at least 1980 there has been a general deforestation of newly planted trees in central Africa for the drying of tobacco. In 1984 there was a symbolic tree-burning ceremony by the Africans at the World Conference on Smoking and Health to highlight this irony. The irony continues to be ignored.

What is becoming more and more amazing is that the tobacco industry continues to argue the evidence against the ill effects of tobacco smoking. No other private organisation would have the gall to dispute any health consequence so well documented. No one would dispute the World Health Organisation. What unqualified individual would argue that, for example, the infection control instigated by the WHO for tuberculosis, the malarias and other infectious diseases was incorrect. What individual would believe themselves better qualified than the WHO? It seems those in the industry do. They feel themselves so far above the scientific evidence that they are willing to take court action to sustain their income. For after all this is what it is all about. These same individuals will wear seatbelts for their safety and the safety of their children, will drink fluoridated water for their teeth and take antibiotics if they have an infection. They see no irony in this. It is only due to the early entry of tobacco into our culture that this situation is even taken seriously today. There would never be a legitimisation of a heroin or cocaine industry today. No one can envisage a company manufacturing heroin, packaging it and selling it over the counter at our local supermarkets, as tobacco is today. The mere fact that arguments arrive in courts of law show that we as a society have not yet the sophistication to treat these industries with the contempt they deserve.

What to do if you can't this time

It may now be that a smoker, having learnt about smoking and nicotine addiction, and attempted to quit, has given it all up and lost the plot. There are many smokers who attempt to quit and do so for a time, 'forget' they can't have Just One and go back to full-on smoking.

Is that the end of it all?

If you have relapsed do not despair!

We know that it may take a smoker three or four serious attempts to quit till it is finally all behind them. Very recent data collected at our Clinic suggests that the older a smoker is the *more* likely they are to quit. The older smoker seems either to have had more experience and has learned to use that past experience or it may be that they are less influenced by social pressures to smoke and more by the social pressures not to. Do not, however, wait till you are too old. Every learning experience adds to the ability to quit permanently. Use each experience of how you coped, and what you can and cannot do to improve things for a future attempt. Never throw your hands up and think that it is all to difficult. Some smokers may think that it is simply not in their hands and will search for a 'magic bullet' to cure them. In the end, the giving up of this substance is in the capacity of everyone if their's is a great enough wish to carry it out. It is hoped that in the future more and more reputable techniques and aids will become available for help, and that with better education there will be more sympathy for the addicted smoker.

Further reading

Richard Bergland, *The Fabric of Mind*, Penguin Books, Ringwood, 1985

Garry Egger and Rosemary Stanton, *Gut Buster*, Allen & Unwin, Sydney, 1992

Victor Frankl, *Man's Search for Meaning*, Hodder & Stoughton, London, 1959

V. G. Keirnan, *Tobacco: A History*, Hutchinson Radius, London, 1991

Jean Lennane, *Alcohol: The National Hangover*, Allen & Unwin, Sydney, 1992

Peter Taylor, *Smoke Ring: The Politics of Tobacco*, Bodley Head, London, 1984

U.S. Surgeon General's Reports, 1975 onward. Available through most libraries